When Your Neurons Dance

As an Emergency Medicine consultant in one of the busiest departments in the UK, Dr Jonny Acheson loved his job. Fuelled by adrenaline, he treated and cared for some of the sickest patients who came through the doors.

In 2016, when he was 41, he was diagnosed with Parkinson's, a progressive neurological condition for which there is no cure.

He found it increasingly difficult to multitask in his fast-paced world. The environment that he thrived in made his symptoms worse. Parkinson's challenged his professional identity as an emergency doctor, and he didn't know what to do.

When Your Neurons Dance is about how he is adapting over time with support around him – how he looked to the past to help him in the present, embracing change as new doors opened both inside and outside medicine.

Ultimately as a doctor practising with Parkinson's, he found a way to give back, despite a condition that always takes away.

When Your Neurons Dance

A STORY OF A DOCTOR WITH PARKINSON'S DISEASE

Jonny Acheson

CRC Press
Taylor & Francis Group
Boca Raton London New York

CRC Press is an imprint of the
Taylor & Francis Group, an **informa** business

Designed cover image: Freepik

First edition published 2026
by CRC Press
2385 NW Executive Center Drive, Suite 320, Boca Raton FL 33431

and by CRC Press
4 Park Square, Milton Park, Abingdon, Oxon, OX14 4RN

CRC Press is an imprint of Taylor & Francis Group, LLC

© 2026 Jonny Acheson

ISBN: 978-1-032-98807-8 (hbk)
ISBN: 978-1-032-98997-6 (pbk)
ISBN: 978-1-003-60067-1 (ebk)

DOI: 10.1201/9781003600671

Typeset in Times LT Std
by Apex CoVantage, LLC

For Heather, Ben and Anna, with all my love.

Contents

Forewords

Jonny Acheson is a natural storyteller, telling this story of his life with great humour, passion and insight. In this book, he shares his life, his work and the challenges of living with Parkinson's. He is an inspiration in so many ways – as a doctor, friend and ambassador for all those living with Parkinson's.

He describes how he joined social media in 2018 to raise awareness of Parkinson's. That's how he and I came across each other, following each other on Twitter (now X) as we both had an interest in Parkinson's. We had not yet met in person when he messaged me one day to ask my advice about recovery from an injury he'd sustained at the Parkinson's Football European Cup in 2019. I also had the privilege of previewing his artwork depicting various Parkinson's symptoms in cartoons. I especially love the one he has done of the word 'exercise' (well, I would – I'm a physiotherapist!). We finally met at a Parkinson's-related event, and he has inspired me ever since.

Jonny's story is a fascinating insight into his early years and his family history in Northern Ireland, his journey into Emergency Medicine and the impact on his life and his family of being given a diagnosis of young onset Parkinson's. Jonny tells his story with humour and throughout the book his passion for sport, especially football (but not golf!) is clear. Indeed, I now know a lot more about football than I did before I read the book!

This book is in part an insight into Jonny's life and experiences, but it is also a helpful source of information and advice for managing Parkinson's symptoms – both for those living with it and for the health professionals working in the field of Parkinson's. Jonny is an ambassador and a motivator, and he raises the importance of people with Parkinson's being given Parkinson's medication on time (it's a time critical medication). He has built up connections with others living with Parkinson's – especially those with young onset Parkinson's – and describes how the NHS Professionals Living with Parkinson's Group came into being and how they have championed the importance of Time Critical Medication. He shares with us the excitement of the evening that they won a (very well-deserved) *Health Service Journal* award for their work so well that I felt I was there!

This book will make you laugh out loud at times (see the description of his encounter with a Japanese toilet) and warm your heart (see the appendix with his daughter's account of her Dad having Parkinson's). If you currently know nothing about Parkinson's, you will be well informed after reading this book; if you are living with Parkinson's, you will be encouraged; if you are working with people with Parkinson's, it will inform and challenge you – especially regarding the importance of people with Parkinson's getting their medication on time.

The epilogue shows where Jonny's strength comes from – and how he has come through many difficult times and challenges. He shares with us where his hope is set. It is a privilege to work alongside Jonny (on the Parkinson's Excellence Network), to be his friend and to have had this insight into his world.

Fiona Lindop MBE
Specialist Physiotherapist in Parkinson's
Clinical Leadership Team Therapy Lead at the Parkinson's Excellence Network

Since our diagnoses of Parkinson's back in 2016 Jonny and I have shared the highs and lows of life with this progressive neurological condition. We are both anxious not to be defined by it, but instead to use our influence as healthcare professionals and our passion for clinical excellence to drive sustainable improvements in Parkinson's care.

In Jonny's inspiring memoirs, we learn of his journey as a medic, son, husband, father and colleague, through the complex world of Parkinson's. He openly shares, through various lenses, how his drive to be the best version of himself, his love of sport, his faith, his determination to maintain his wellness and his extraordinary creative talents have not only enabled him to rise to the challenges that life has seemingly indiscriminately thrown at him but also to advocate for and influence care of the wider Parkinson's community.

For the reader there is a huge privilege in being given insight into this exceptional human being's world; his humble and humanistic style guaranteeing an inclusive read, grounded by life's harsh reality. Educational, honest and motivational . . . a must read for all members of the Parkinson's community and beyond.

Clare Addison
NHS Healthcare Professional Living with Parkinson's

Preface

As the dawn chorus sang, I started to type every day as daylight began to appear. The words kept coming and in the quietness at the start of the day, I could visualise the chapters with clarity. People with Parkinson's need time and this was when I had the most.

The first book describing Parkinson's, published in 1817, was titled 'An Essay on The Shaking Palsy.' Since then, many books have been written on the subject, authored by doctors, healthcare professionals, scientists and people living with the condition alike, all bringing their perspectives.

This book is different as it is written by an NHS doctor with Parkinson's. It explores the dynamic of how as a patient I had to learn to live with Parkinson's, to enable me to keep practising. The truth is at diagnosis. I didn't know very much about Parkinson's but with education came the ability to adapt. With adaption came acceptance.

As a society we like to commentate on the extraordinary and that is necessary. It is the extraordinary that inspires, lifts the bar on possibility and gives rise to invention. But this is an effort to dissect the ordinary. A lived experience, common to millions of people, in the hope of challenging how we think about the ordinary to transform the everyday.

Acknowledgements

There are many people to thank for helping this book get to the stage of being published. Thanks to Miranda, Paige and Reuben at Taylor and Francis for believing that there was a story to be written and for being so patient as the task was undertaken.

Thanks to the entire Parkinson's community. It was simply impossible to mention everyone who has helped me along my journey to date, from the online community, the charitable sector and those living with it every day.

Thanks to the University Hospitals of Leicester NHS Trust and the whole ED team. It is a blessing to not only be able to continue working but to enjoy doing so and that is due to you all. In particular to my line managers Mandeep and Julie D for your unwavering support in enabling the necessary adjustments. Thanks also to the Parkinson's Excellence Network for the work you do and for letting me contribute to it in some small way as we continue to improve the care for people with Parkinson's.

To my healthcare team both past and present who have managed my condition to enable function nine years later – far more than I dared hope.

Thanks to all who took the time to read and make suggestions on the early drafts, especially my brother Tim and my Uncle Paul. To my brother Peter for being my fact checker. Thanks also to my support network of friends, extended family and church.

To my dad for showing me that through adversity and trials that there is a life to be lived and to my mum for her encouraging words and her unwavering ability to keep going. That no matter what life throws at you, you have a choice with how you respond. To my in-laws and my brother-in-law and his family – you all have helped me immeasurably in more ways than you will ever know.

Finally to Heather, Ben and Anna for your patience and love.

Heather you know me so well that you were able to help put into words what I was really trying to say and to give a glimpse into our lives with Parkinson's.

About the Author

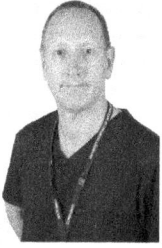

Jonny Acheson is currently an NHS Emergency Medicine consultant who advocates to increase the quality of care for people with Parkinson's when they are in hospital. He, alongside fellow NHS professionals living and working with Parkinson's, has put Time Critical Medication on the national agenda working alongside Parkinson's UK. He is currently the Director of Engagement at the Parkinson's Excellence Network, a post he has held since 2022. He studied medicine at Queens University Belfast and subsequently worked in Emergency Departments in both Northern Ireland and the East Midlands. He dabbles in letter art to create short films and sketches to educate about Parkinson's. He has exhibited in Leicester, Barcelona and Paris.

He lives in Leicestershire with his wife and two children.

Author's Note

The stories in this book are written from my memory of events that happened in real time. The names and locations of patients if mentioned at all have been changed to protect their confidentiality. I am grateful to the NHS staff, members of the Parkinson's Excellence Network and the people with Parkinson's who have allowed me to use their real names.

CHAPTER 1

The Long Walk

I had entered the building countless times during the past twelve years so there was a welcome sense of familiarity, but it did nothing to settle the knot in my stomach. On this occasion, I wasn't there in a professional capacity or calling to visit someone.

In the Leicester General Hospital, all activity branches off the spine of its central corridor which is one hundred and seventy metres long. When the building opened in 1902 it was claimed to be the longest such corridor in England. I'm not sure about the truth of that claim but I do know that when you enter at one end it's usually impossible to see to the other. Equipment, patients on trolleys and a bustling array of staff and visitors always obscure the horizon.

People hurried past me without eye contact. That was normal. Staff were busy and probably had somewhere they were meant to be half an hour ago. This wasn't a stroll in the park where there is time to stop for chat about the weather. This was the NHS in full flow, a flow that I had been part of every day for the past seventeen years. But this time I was part of a different current. For the first time the corridor felt long and, in the silence, I reached for the hand of Heather, my wife.

There are always people lost in hospitals. They can be seen hovering near one of those maps which tells you where you are but not where you need to be or observed rustling through the bundle of papers which accompany every appointment letter. That day I knew exactly where I was going. I could navigate my way without assistance. The signs above departments were in a language I understood. Even faces in the busy corridor were identifiable and yet the landscape felt new. I was about to understand that being lost doesn't always involve maps or directions.

Eventually, even one hundred and seventy metres ends, and I arrived at my destination. To be honest if I hadn't known where I was going it would have been easily missed. Earlier Heather and I had walked past the Diabetes Centre with its white polished entrance and painted green leaves that looked like they were growing from the floor up the side of the doors to the roof. We had peered through one of the large glass doors at the entrance. It was inviting, accessible and warm. We don't as healthcare professionals always recognise the importance of surroundings. Indeed, when you are used to the frontline and dealing with emergencies, they can often seem rather superfluous considerations. But that afternoon I discovered that when you are feeling vulnerable, uncertain and anxious, they make the world of difference.

DOI: 10.1201/9781003600671-1

Our destination was marked by a small, unremarkable sign three-quarters of the way up the wall that simply said 'Neurology Outpatients.' It is amazing the details that we notice, even in moments of mental turmoil. There was a standard outer navy door which had seen better days. It was dented in several places, with a 'Keep Clear, Fire Exit' sticker on it and two exclamation marks. This led immediately into a closet-sized space measuring six feet by four feet where we encountered yet another door, unmarked and painted grey. In that moment, it felt akin to being in an airlock, confined between two doors separating two worlds. My anxiety heightened. This wasn't a wardrobe that led to Narnia, but it was a step into the unknown.

I opened the second door to find a standard run-of-the-mill reception with high-backed green leather-covered chairs and bare walls that looked in desperate need of a lick of paint. I booked in and turned to assess the waiting room. There was a lady, sitting in a wheelchair, in the front row. Quickly noticing a marked tremor in her left arm, it was easy to identify why she was at the neurology clinic. But I could see nothing obvious to explain the attendance of the man in the blue-checked shirt three chairs behind.

From the earliest days of medical training, we are taught to observe, to be constantly on the lookout for those clinical signs, often unrecognised by the patient themselves, which act as markers for disease. It's impossible to walk down the street and not at least unconsciously spot the people who have pathology. We are trained until it becomes instinctive. But as I scanned the waiting room, I suddenly became mindful of what others might be thinking about me. That afternoon I felt like a specimen on the slide of a microscope, every detail under scrutiny.

I was anxious deciding where to sit, which with hindsight seems ridiculous. The waiting room was not full and there were lots of empty chairs. But I was disorientated because familiarity lay behind the clinic door. If I'm honest I was also very conscious about bumping into someone I knew. At this stage, in addition to my consultant role in the Emergency Department (ED) I also had a role arranging final examinations at the medical school. Both meant I was in regular contact with colleagues across all medical specialities. I did not want to have to explain to people that I worked with why I was sitting in the clinic waiting room as a patient.

Walking to the back row of the waiting room I strategically sat down on the closest chair to clinic number four, the room I knew the neurologist was working out of that day, hoping it would minimise the chances of recognition. I sat and wished there was a magazine to grab but, in keeping with a script from a TV sitcom, almost immediately, one of the hospital's resuscitation officers entered the outpatient area for a routine check of the equipment and drugs in the cardiac arrest trolley. My heart sank. I may have positioned myself in the back row but I wasn't hidden and he soon spotted me. True to the ethos in the NHS of being part of team, he came to say hello. We chatted for a few minutes but by the time he left my anxiety levels had rocketed further.

The waiting was the hardest part. The sixty seconds it took to go around the circumference of the clock on the wall felt like an eternity but eventually the clinic door opened and the neurologist, whom I knew, beckoned me into his office. I repeated the story I had told my GP a week ago, the same one which had replayed in my mind countless times since.

Several weeks earlier we had been spending Friday evening with friends and their families. It was noisy, fun and full of energy. At one point, my friend decided to demonstrate a move he had learnt at his daughter's Bollywood dance class. We all jumped up off the sofa to have a go at the 'changing the lightbulb' dance. He put both his hands up in the air in front of him, the left one slightly higher than the right one. (In all honesty, I don't think it mattered if you put your right one higher than the left). He then proceeded to rhythmically rotate his left and right wrists. Anna, my daughter, picked it up immediately but as I attempted to copy, I realised that no matter how hard I tried, I was not able to rotate my left wrist at speed compared to the right one. I internally instructed my wrist to move faster but all the encouragement and willpower in the world didn't have any effect. It bothered me. I showed Heather and her concern did little to settle my own growing unease. Over the incoming days, I tried again and again but it stayed slow, and nothing would speed it up. In my gut I knew something was wrong and that I needed to see someone about it.

I made an appointment with my GP as soon as I could. She was amazing that day. The door of the waiting room opened, and she called my name with a smile. I followed her into one of the consultation rooms, sat down and immediately acknowledged there was something wrong. 'I can't rotate my left wrist very quickly,' I told her. She listened patiently, carefully enquiring about other symptoms. 'Tiredness,' I remarked, but there was nothing unexpected in that. We were heading into exam season at the medical school and work in the ED was relentlessly busy at this time of the year. Heather pointed out that I occasionally seemed to trip over my foot when walking. The GP then examined me and confirmed indirectly that there was something wrong by referring me for an urgent CT scan and neurology review. I have always wanted to ask her if she knew what the diagnosis was when she referred me that day. I suspect she did.

Back in clinic, the neurologist summarised the symptoms and enquired about others. He then asked me to walk across the length of the waiting room. I often do this with my patients, but I had never had to do it myself. I was determined not to scuff my left foot. I wanted to walk seamlessly in front of the neurologist and so I took it slowly. It didn't take long to cross and come back. Completing the task without incident, I exhaled with relief that I hadn't scuffed my left foot. I smiled at the neurologist and he smiled back but in an awkward, non-reassuring way that evaded eye contact. I could sense something wasn't quite right and sat down in the clinic chair. 'You don't swing your left arm very much when you walk.' This was the second sign that something in my left arm wasn't working properly. 'I'm going to order a DAT scan.'

Now, I had attended most lectures as a medical student at Queen's University Belfast, but I do not recall anyone mentioning what a DAT scan was. I looked at Heather with a slightly confused look. She, as a trainee in old age psychiatry, knew exactly the implication, but I was in the dark.

'He doesn't know why you are doing that,' she said gently, leaning forward to catch the eye of the neurologist. He acknowledged what she had said and paused. Then looking directly at me said, 'I am very sorry to have to tell you, Jonny, it is likely you have idiopathic Parkinson's disease.' It was 14:24 on 4th April 2016.

I distinctly recall being taught during my medical training that people will forget around ninety percent of the information they are given during a medical consultation. Certainly, after hearing the words Parkinson's disease only a few key phrases broke through. I heard him tell me that it was at a mild stage and I remember being surprised at his explanation that seventy percent of my brain cells had already died at diagnosis. That didn't sound mild to me but to be honest most of what he said was drowned out by a cacophony of internal questions. Why did I not work it out? How could I have been so blindsided?

I suspect how anyone responds to a diagnosis is partly influenced by their personality and character. I'm by nature all about the practicalities – I like to get things done, to sort and fix. With reflection, I realised at this initial stage that my first concern was not to understand what was wrong, or why it had happened. That would follow very quickly. But in the immediate aftermath, as the shock of the diagnosis registered and the implications hit me, I wanted to know one thing above all others.

I spoke with directness, 'You need to tell me what I should do.'

He went on to suggest that exercise would help my symptoms; but he didn't expand on what type or how much, and that I needed to keep my stress levels as low as possible. He instructed me to inform the Driving Vehicle Licensing Agency (DVLA) and my insurance company about my diagnosis and explained that whilst there was no cure there were medications effective at masking the symptoms. He suggested that I didn't presently need levodopa but did prescribe a tablet called rasagiline. Finally, he advised that it would be a good idea to take some time off work as this was a big shock and not one that I was expecting to hear. He wasn't wrong.

Simply Complex

I left the hospital with Heather, on the one hand experiencing a strange sense of detachment as though in a dream, and on the other overwhelmed by waves of emotion confirming that I wasn't. In that moment I desperately wanted to be anywhere else and as I sat in the passenger seat of the car if I could have pressed an ejector button I would have done so.

I also felt confused. When I had arrived at the hospital, I was prepared for several outcomes, but Parkinson's was not one of them. It just hadn't crossed my mind as a possibility. Twenty years earlier at medical school I had first encountered Parkinson's during a forty-five-minute lecture on chronic neurological conditions. I thought I knew how to diagnose it and yet it seemed I had missed it in myself. I understood it as a condition affecting older people but here I was, with a diagnosis at only forty-one years of age. I could describe the pathology, but I had no knowledge how I was now to live with it.

I desperately retreated to the depths of my memory attempting to recall the spider diagrams of revision notes. Tremor, stiffness, slowness and old were words which quickly sprung to mind but none of them resonated with my present experience. I didn't fit my own mental picture of Parkinson's and beyond the looping soundtrack 'I have Parkinson's disease' I felt lost.

The drive home was a familiar one. We passed the primary school where Ben and Anna were happy and secure in their classrooms. How on earth were we going to tell them? When should we tell them? Should we even tell them? The questions started and didn't stop. So many questions without answers; like breakers on a beach they rolled, one after another, each knocking me off balance.

Past, present and future all suddenly looked different and wherever my mind travelled questions appeared. We passed a church, and I wondered if I would be able to walk my daughter down the aisle in the years to come. We continued past the golf course, and I considered whether Parkinson's was the reason I kept hitting the ball to the right at every hole. (Seven years later when I was having a golf lesson it became clear that it wasn't Parkinson's, it was just that I wasn't any good at golf.) By the time we reached home I was utterly shattered.

I turned the key to unlock the front door just as I had done hundreds of times before. On automatic pilot, I took off my coat, reached up and placed it on the top, furthest

DOI: 10.1201/9781003600671-2

left, coat peg. (I always use the same peg. I have no idea why. Perhaps it is simply one less decision out of the countless that need to be made every day.) As I did so I caught sight of the lower coat peg rack, recently put up so the kids could put away their own coats. Two weeks before I had managed to get down on my knees and drill two holes in the wall, aligned at the correct distance, to enable me to fix it. It is amazing how the mundane can become significant. In that moment a flicker of determination ignited. I did not want to give up drilling holes just yet.

Entering the kitchen, the familiar surroundings of home felt odd in a way that I knew had nothing to do with bricks and mortar. Three hours earlier I had left as Jonny, husband and dad, but now I wasn't sure who I was. The reality is that I had been living with Parkinson's disease (PD), unbeknown to me or my family, for longer than I had thought. Seventy percent of my dopamine-producing brain cells had not just died overnight. This had been a slow burn over many years and had gone undetected until a tipping point was reached. It's a cunning creeper of a disease causing a dopamine deficiency which doesn't stop just because you have been diagnosed. Looking back over the proceeding eighteen months from a new perspective, I began to acknowledge that signs suggesting something was wrong had been there, we just hadn't joined the dots. I had been distant and emotionless and gone from being a hands-on husband and dad to someone with little interest who kept falling asleep on the sofa even before the kids had gone to bed. And it wasn't just evenings. There had been occasions during the day when I had just needed to put my arms down on my desk and rest my head as I fought to keep my eyes open. I would fall asleep at the noisiest swimming gala with hundreds of children screaming encouragement to their club teammates and, by the time the last swimmer dived into the water for the relay, I could be found with my head bowed drifting in and out of a state of consciousness. I even managed to find myself falling asleep at the King Power Stadium, home of Leicester City Football Club, while thirty-two thousand fans belted out 'Jamie Vardy's having a party.' And for anyone who knows me well, falling asleep at a football match was an alarm bell.

I felt guilty and to a degree embarrassed that we hadn't identified the diagnosis earlier. I think these emotions were especially prominent because of our jobs. During medical training much of what we learn is undertaken in abstract. We acquire knowledge of different conditions but usually in isolation from patient stories and lives, and the result is that we end up conceptualising diseases predominantly in terms of physical signs and symptoms as if we can somehow always segregate and independently assess what is biological. But the reality is we are all holistic beings with social, psychological and spiritual dimensions, and identifying what is biological is sometimes not as straightforward as we like to believe. This is especially true when non-specific symptoms are being considered. I was fatigued but I was working a busy job, whilst undertaking a master's degree and looking after a young family, so that didn't seem particularly unusual.

Slumping into my favourite wicker chair in the kitchen I closed my eyes hoping everything would revert to normal when I opened them, but of course it didn't.

This diagnosis was a seismic event, which had, in an instant, changed our life. The incoming months would necessitate a slow process of clearing debris and reconstruction but in the immediate aftershock necessity was paramount. Top of our priority list were the kids and we understood that regardless of how we were feeling, the day-to-day running of family life somehow had to continue. Drinking a welcome cup of coffee, Heather and I discussed what we should tell Ben and Anna.

We have always operated an open book policy with our kids, encouraging them to ask any question, any time, and we quickly concluded that this situation should not be any different. They had both been aware I was visiting a doctor at the hospital so we knew the conversation would be easy to raise but we had no idea how to explain a disease, first described as a neurological syndrome over two hundred years ago and which has over forty different symptoms, to a six- and a ten-year-old. We agreed on a simple approach and later that evening told them in a way that we hoped they could grasp. I simply explained that I didn't have enough chemicals in the part of my brain that made me move normally or be myself, and it was called Parkinson's.

Ben immediately asked, 'Will you always be the same?'

How do you begin to answer a question you can't answer yourself? I stalled. If I replied no, then he would worry, and it would inevitably lead to further difficult questions. If I answered yes, it would have been a lie.

Children need to feel loved and secure and have the freedom to be children as long as they can. No one wants them to grow up too fast. But that must be balanced sometimes with the cold and harsh reality of life. In the end I didn't directly answer the question but told him the truth; I didn't know. I reassured him that it was presently very mild and reminded him that whatever else changed I would still be his dad. He then asked, 'Will we still be able to go and watch Leicester City when they are playing at home?' Children have a wonderful ability to ground you in the normal. 'Of course,' I said mustering a smile I didn't feel. That seemed to be acceptable and pacified any need for any further questions.

As I turned to Anna I observed a more inquisitive look on her face. She is a child who has never been content to accept things at face value, the child who always asks 'Why?' If I could have looked directly into her brain, I would have seen the cogs whirring at a rapid pace with steam rising from them. She simply asked, 'What made it happen?' When I replied, 'No one really knows Anna,' she turned quick as a flash and enquired, 'Why not?'

Drowning in a sea of questions immediately after diagnosis, my first instinct, much like Anna's, was to seek answers and explanations. I too wanted to understand what had caused this. Why me? Why now? Why Parkinson's? were questions I suspect everyone asks at some point. As a clinician I pored over the scientific literature but in the end was left with more questions and few answers. Given my young age of onset there was a long, nervous wait of many weeks for the results of genetic testing to see if this would shed some light. It didn't. Although they provided some reassurance, they didn't bring peace of mind.

At present there is so much about Parkinson's that we don't understand, and among the many questions that had flooded to the surface some had sprung from existential curiosity. The first step in my journey of adaptation was to seek wisdom to separate those questions to which I could find answers, from those which, no matter how hard I tried, would remain cloaked in mystery. This was important to conserve energy and to direct resources towards endeavours which would yield profit rather than leave me feeling frustrated. Ultimately, I had to find peace with the fact that some questions, at least for now, have no answers. I also had to accept that the absence of answers did not mean an absence of choice. I didn't choose Parkinson's but could choose to release the pause button it had pressed on my life. However, enacting our choices is not always as easy as making them. The worry and fear of the unknown can occasionally feel overwhelming, and I needed help. I am fortunate that there was plenty around in the form of my family, friends and charities but ultimately, I found it most in my faith in Christ and my belief that the events of my life are not located in random chaos but in a loving God. This isn't a book about faith, however; adapting to disease involves all aspects of who we are. I didn't need all the answers to move forward, I just needed the answer that would help me find the first step.

———————————

The weeks following passed in a haze of emotional exhaustion as we broke the diagnosis to the broader family and friends and for a while there was little time to properly process anything. Eventually, however, the initial aftershocks began to diminish and there were periods of quiet in which I could begin to move beyond surviving the day, to contemplate the path ahead. But the task that confronted me was harder than I had anticipated. It was not just a case of reconstructing what had been flattened. The diagnosis had changed the landscape, and I found myself rebuilding in a foreign land – one I didn't really comprehend. I realised that before anything else I had to understand and familiarise myself with my new surroundings. My mind drifted back to that university lecture almost twenty years earlier where I had learnt about Parkinson's. The dissonance between what I remembered and my personal experience still bothered me.

Keen to find out more I visited my local library to see if I could find a book on Parkinson's that wasn't a medical textbook. There was only one on the shelf. Intrigued, I removed it and found a quiet corner to sit down. It was in good condition which meant it was either a new book or no one had ever taken it out. When I opened the front of it and turned to read the first page, a simple Venn diagram caught my attention. It had three interlinked circles, one was physical health, one was mental health and one was social health. I read the text underneath that said, 'If you have all three of these in balance you will give yourself the best chance of living well with Parkinson's in your life every day.' However, at this stage I did not need lofty aspirations (though I could recognise their truth) but practical solutions that would enable me to find that balance. So, I returned home and did what most people now do after receiving a diagnosis – I hit Google search. What I discovered surprised me.

Davis Phinney was an American cyclist who competed at the Olympics and the Tour de France. He was diagnosed with Parkinson's at the age of forty-one. He and his wife Connie set up the Davis Phinney Foundation for Parkinson's, with the ethos of helping people live as well as they could every day. This struck a chord with me. I knew despite advances in understanding that there wasn't a cure around the corner any time soon, so discovering and putting into practice ways in which I could live well and optimise function seemed reasonable.

Their information felt personable and relatable. I wasn't an Olympic cyclist, and I had never cycled in the Tour De France, but I was forty-one, married, raising a young family and working hard in my career. Helpfully the foundation had a book called *Every Victory Counts* that could be ordered as a digital download. First published in 2010 it focuses on the concept of proactive self-care and a holistic approach to the management of Parkinson's. The word proactive immediately grabbed my attention. When you are diagnosed with a progressive, degenerating condition there is an immediate sense of losing control. But the word proactive suggested I could regain some of that control that, in some measure, I could get ahead of the ball. There may not be a cure but there were things I could do to help. I felt I could really relate to a mindset that embraced making changes to the way I lived with Parkinson's, rather than Parkinson's dictating and calling the shots. I took the plunge and downloaded the three hundred pages plus PDF file.

I was never a reader. Heather could devour four or five books on a week-long holiday whereas I barely managed one, but I couldn't put this one down. It was packed to the rafters, bulging at the seams with information that just kept flowing. It was obvious I had movement symptoms on my left side manifesting in the slow rotation of my wrist and the scuffing of my left foot. But I began identifying other symptoms that I hadn't recognised as part of Parkinson's.

In the months before diagnosis, I was needing to stop around fifteen minutes into every run because of pain in my right knee. It suddenly made sense that if I wasn't walking properly due to stiffness and rigidity on my left side then I wasn't running properly either. I was putting extra strain on my right knee when I ran, overcompensating for the deficits on my left side.

My absence of smell was also I discovered due to Parkinson's. I can smell the scent of a rose or Chanel No. 5 but little else. It's not a symptom you always notice. I have since learnt that loss of smell can be one of the earliest symptoms to develop in Parkinson's.

The big picture became clearer as different pieces of the jigsaw fell into place and I immediately began to feel better. I felt a huge sense of relief when I discovered that my tendency to fall asleep everywhere was pathological fatigue, a very common symptom of Parkinson's. I wasn't disinterested, I wasn't overworked, I wasn't burning the candle at both ends or stressed; I simply did not have enough dopamine in the tank to keep functioning. I was like a car that was running out of petrol, or like a battery running out of charge.

Reading can be a great way to navigate information. Having someone directly explain this vastly intricate and complex condition in such a simple and easy-to-follow way was a great help. I was able to take time and absorb information at my own pace, re-reading things as I needed. What helped me was the information from Davis Phinney, in part because of similarities in our story, but there is a wealth of helpful and practical information out there. Another good place to start is the charity Parkinson's UK. What matters is that you find information you can relate to and if your first attempt doesn't quite help then I would encourage you to keep persevering.

At this stage I was like a sponge, keen to absorb as much information as possible realising that every new piece of knowledge was clearing the fog of confusion that had descended the instant I heard the words Parkinson's disease. Each piece of information, gathered over weeks, was valuable, but arguably the most helpful for me was to grasp the distinction between two broad groups of symptoms in PD – the motor symptoms and the non-motor ones.

I watched a YouTube video called 'The Parkinson's You Don't See: Cognitive and Non-Motor Symptoms,' which was one of the most enlightening and educational twenty-six minutes I had spent thus far. The motor symptoms are those I had quickly recalled – the ones most people associate with Parkinson's, shuffling, slowness, stiffness, tremor. The non-motor symptoms tend to be less visible, are often more disabling and are less well understood by the public and healthcare professionals.

Anxiety is a prominent non-motor symptom, and it had become an unwelcome friend. Before Parkinson's I would have described myself as relaxed, chilled and easy-going. But not anymore. It remains one of my more disabling symptoms, but it made a huge difference to understand that it was part of my presentation.

I think we often underestimate the effect of validating patient experiences. When you experience symptoms which are distressing but attributable, it does not diminish their impact, but it does avoid the additional distress of trying to make sense of them. Removing them from the realm of the subjective into objectivity is profoundly reassuring and saves restless nights wondering if it's all in your imagination. It makes it easier to communicate your experience and finally when you understand the cause of symptoms it does of course provide a basis for starting to manage them.

My anxiety started with difficulty making the simplest of decisions – like who to pick for my fantasy football team, paralysed by fear of making a wrong decision. This was especially heightened in unfamiliar situations, but in the months leading up to my diagnosis I had also started to avoid large crowds. I hated the feeling of being confined in a crowded space, and on several occasions this had escalated into a panic attack. One such episode occurred during a family weekend trip to London, the week before I saw my GP. As I walked down the platform at St Pancras having disembarked from the train, I observed a swarm of people at the ticket barrier up ahead. It was like we were all tins on a production line all massed together. I didn't like the feeling of my personal space being invaded. The feeling of claustrophobia intensified when I was separated from the rest of my family. As the barrier approached my anxiety heightened and I felt I was going to pass out. By the time I scanned my ticket it was as though the world had become unreal. I was hyperventilating and it wasn't until I walked through to the other side and the crowds began to disperse that I felt relief.

I had also found myself increasingly leaving the Leicester City matches early to avoid the crowds at the final whistle. As soon as the clock hit eighty-six minutes I was on my feet, any fatigue I was feeling temporarily dissipated by the desire to exit before everyone else. Ben hated leaving early and I hated disappointing him but neither the guilt nor fear of missing out were sufficient to overcome the anxiety. Walking back to the car we would occasionally hear a massive cheer. Leicester had either extended their lead, equalised or scored a winner and we had missed it. We now follow the end of the game listening to BBC Leicester, until the referee has blown the full-time whistle, but it's not quite the same when you are walking in the opposite direction.

There has been just one occasion when we didn't leave before the match finished. It was a bright Saturday afternoon, four weeks after my diagnosis, and no one was leaving early that day. Leicester had just won the 2015–2016 Premier League title, a feat that will go down in football folklore, and we had been fortunate to be with them every home game. No one could quite believe it and the atmosphere in the city during those few weeks was unforgettable. As I entered the turnstiles for the final time that infamous season, I felt more optimistic. After four weeks off work and a lot of reading, help and support from my family and friends, I had begun to find solid ground beneath my feet. The turmoil of the aftermath had subsided and though I was still navigating a new landscape the beginnings of reconstruction had started to emerge.

During the post-match celebrations, the Leicester City manager Claudio Ranieri introduced the famous Italian tenor, Andrea Bocelli. Cheered by more than thirty thousand fans he started to sing 'Time to Say Goodbye' and as he did so all the emotion from the past four weeks hit me. As the tears ran down my face it felt like I was saying goodbye to my old life and turning a page to start a new chapter. That was the first time I cried, but it wouldn't be the last. The path ahead was uncertain but I had found my first step. Written large on the blank page of the new chapter was a phrase that would help shape the weeks ahead. Do what you can. The first goal I set was two and a half hours of high-intensity exercise each week. The challenge was how to achieve it.

This Bike Is on Me

Parkinson's is a progressive condition characterised by continuous change, so adaptability is an essential skill. However, change is not unique to Parkinson's. Nature depends on water, carbon and nitrogen cycling. There are tides and seasons, death and birth, invention and decline. Change is a constant in all our lives, and we are continually processing and managing it. Most of the time it happens imperceptibly, beyond our sense of awareness, but when change is unwelcome or imposed then it tends to make its presence known. In such circumstances, the initial instinct is to mount resistance.

In the weeks immediately following diagnosis, my priority was to ensure I was doing everything possible to limit the advance of change. There were several dimensions to this but the one with most consensus and evidence and which I could implement quickly was exercise.

_____

Sport played a pivotal role throughout my childhood and teens. I suspect it was encouraged by my parents as a means of managing my high levels of energy. However, the truth is that I needed little persuading. I loved the competitive element, the drive that pushes for the win, the buzz that comes from enduring that ten seconds longer or running that one km farther.

I remember as an eleven-year-old child receiving a football net for Christmas. It was by far my favourite present that year and quickly led to a new daily routine. As soon as I returned from school, I would drop my school bag at the back door, shout to mum that everything was good and run straight up to my bedroom. I hurriedly changed into my football kit and, abandoning my uniform in a heap on the floor, hurtled back downstairs, straight through the kitchen, grabbing from mum's hand whatever snack was on offer and into the back garden. No matter the weather I would be outside within five minutes scanning for the football.

It was never long until it was found and positioned on a carefully determined spot in the top right-hand corner of the grass, leaving just enough room for a run-up and enabling me to plant my right foot. Taking aim, I would attempt to bend the ball around the trunk of the large apple tree, in the middle of the garden, and into the top left-hand corner of the net. Whatever the outcome, successful or not, I collected the ball and repeated the whole process. The same ritual, time after time, day after day.

DOI: 10.1201/9781003600671-3

They say practice makes perfect but there is no such thing as perfection in sport, and there were frequent occasions when I couldn't stop the ball from rising, flying over the bar and rebounding off the kitchen window. I would watch in slow motion, holding my breath, as the pane of single-glazing glass wobbled like jelly. The thud always acted to alert mum, and it wasn't long before she was knocking the window and wagging her finger from side to side. Her communication was clear; practice was finished for the day.

I not only loved playing football, I also loved watching it. Local football, club football, international football – it didn't really matter. But what I enjoyed more than anything was watching Northern Ireland play.

Northern Ireland football has had its fair share of ups and downs over the years and it isn't always an easy watch. However, there are a few special moments. One of them was the 1982 World Cup. It was during the Troubles and Northern Ireland's participation in such a big event had provided several weeks of welcome diversion. (The only time they had previously reached the World Cup finals was in Sweden, in 1958 when they reached the quarter final.) I distinctly remember, as an eight-year-old boy, our whole family sitting on our sofa to watch them take on the mighty hosts Spain. Even mum, who never watched football, had joined us.

We had already played our first two matches, drawing against Yugoslavia and Honduras, so this result was crucial if we hoped to progress. No one gave us a chance. The first half was a quiet affair and as the whistle blew to start the second half, the game was finely balanced. We were just settling back with our customary snack of crisps when Billy Hamilton whipped in a perfect low cross which the Spanish goalkeeper, who was at full stretch, could only palm forwards. Gerry Armstrong, the Northern Ireland number 9, didn't miss the target, and as he smashed it low into the back of the Spanish net, five bodies jumped and wildly celebrated.

By the time we had calmed down, the realisation dawned that there were still another forty minutes to play, which allowed ample time for Spain to equalise. Those minutes felt like an eternity and when the referee blew the final whistle, we could hardly believe they had managed to hold on. The men in green, the underdogs, the team that no one gave a chance, had overcome the odds. They had dug deep to find a way and in doing so pulled off one of the shock results in the history of the whole World Cup. This is the power of sport. Gerry Armstrong went on to forge a career out of that one famous goal and I believed thereafter that anything is possible.

As I moved into my teens, my love of sport diversified to include anything involving a ball. I still loved football but what became more important was the ability to be active. At secondary school, tennis and rugby were added to the mix. I put my kicking foot to use as the number 10 on the school rugby team and exchanged my shin pads for a mouth guard. But in my final year of school, I encountered a problem.

At sixteen I had spent a year living in America on a school exchange programme. The Department of Education rules meant I found myself too old and unable to play for the school in my final year. For the first time in over ten years I was not part of a sporting team. I was frustrated and disappointed and didn't know what to do. The solution arrived unexpectedly.

Early one Saturday morning I heard the doorbell ring. Still tired from a late night before, I made no effort to move from my coffee and left mum to answer. However, the house was not large and so it wasn't long before I could hear the caller enquire whether I was at home. Curiosity led me to abandon my comfort and I wandered into the hall to be greeted by a firm handshake and a warm introduction.

'Hello, I'm Merton and I hear you have a gem of a left foot.' Merton was captain of the 5th XV team at Banbridge Town Rugby Club. They played at Rifle Park whose grounds were less than a mile from our house.

'Would you consider playing rugby for the town this year?' he continued. 'There are matches home and away but don't worry transport is provided and we'll look after you.' I could see no reason to decline.

'Sounds brilliant,' I replied, 'when is the first game?'

He laughed as he replied, 'In about four hours!'

My first game was against a Northern Ireland Police side, then known as the Royal Ulster Constabulary. It was a tight fixture and they were well organised: big and hard to run through. With the scores tied at nine each and only seconds on the clock we won a penalty on the ten-metre line. The choice Merton faced, as captain, was whether to kick or run with the ball. If we kicked for touch that would give the opposition team the throw-in and we would likely lose possession. If we ran we were more likely to run out of time than ground. That left the option of kicking for goal.

Merton looked at me asking, 'Is it too far?'

I thought it probably was but . . . there was quite a strong wind at my back. For a moment doubt hovered and then the love of a challenge kicked in.

'I think I can reach it,' I replied.

I took the ball in my hands and dried it on my shirt. I looked at the referee and indicated that we were going to kick for goal. There was a routine to what followed. I planted my right foot beside the ball and took two large steps backwards then two steps to the right. Slightly hunched, I looked first at the posts, then at the ball as I focused on the exact point I was going to strike.

As the ball rose from the ground, it was straight and on target, gaining height by the second. Both sides watched anxiously as it reached its maximum height trajectory and started to fall. It was going to be close. As the ball struck the crossbar; time stood still, my eyes fixed on the ball. The wind helped it over and we won by twelve points to nine.

In a rugby club, there is a great sense of community; everyone's lives are different, and everyone's weeks are different, yet on a Saturday afternoon none of those matter. For eighty minutes there is a shared objective and collective unity. Bonds are formed on a rectangular pitch with an oblong ball. Fifteen players in fifteen different positions all with a particular job to do.

These recollections demonstrate how physical activity can promote well-being. It develops resilience, encourages perseverance and expands community. However, perhaps most importantly it fosters self-belief and teaches that we don't have to settle for the status quo. Sport never rests where it is. Whether golf, swimming, tennis or running, boundaries are always being pushed to go further, faster, better: raising the bar of expectation to lead us to new realms of possibility. Change is an integral part of sport and success in it depends on finding a balance between pushing limits to improve and recognising limitations to avoid injury. Many of the skills it develops can be extrapolated to help us adapt to change in other domains of life. However, the ignition spark that powers all change is desire. You only succeed in sport if firstly you want to and secondly if you believe it is possible. I had to believe I could kick the goal to achieve it and the same is true in adapting to Parkinson's. You first must want to change.

The benefits of exercise for everyone, with Parkinson's or not, are well known. And yet despite my active participation in sport as a child and my inherent love of it, the harsh truth is that in the ten years before I was diagnosed, I had largely stopped all regular exercise beyond walking with the pram or subsequently playing with the kids in the back garden.

Knowing something is good for us doesn't mean we always do it. Enjoying it doesn't always mean that we make time for it. It isn't always a lack of motivation or ignorance that keeps us inactive, it's often priorities. I had been playing five-a-side football every Monday evening but stopped going the week after my son was born and never restarted. Life just got busier, my priorities changed and exercise fell down the list. There were simply other things that I decided were more important to me at that time. It is amazing how three words, 'You have Parkinson's,' can turn a priority list on its head. They acted as a very loud wake-up call and the necessary spark of desire was re-ignited.

I was never much of a gym person before my diagnosis. It was something I dipped in and out of as I found time or inclination. But four weeks after I was diagnosed, I joined the university gym as I decided this was the best way to ensure exercise became a regular part of my routine. I planned to attend four mornings a week before work: Monday, Tuesday, Wednesday and Friday. I made this a priority and sacrificed breakfast with the family on these days to be at the gym by opening at 6.30 am. It was not easy, but I weighed up the pros and cons and focused on the long-term benefits.

First up was a gym induction: I had attended gym inductions before, but the instructors were usually younger, stronger and more interested in what size of weight I could lift. When I met with Mark it was clear he was different. He listened intently to why I wanted to exercise. He asked when I could exercise and for how long, and he listened to what type of exercise I needed. Over the next sixty minutes he took me on various machines, to determine if I could manage them and to assess my level of fitness. He then took me away from my favoured cardio machines and plotted a strength routine with weights and a stretch and balance routine. In total, I would do forty-five minutes – thirty minutes of cardiovascular fitness on the machines and fifteen minutes on strength and balance. He said one thing to me that day which I have never forgotten – 'Jonny, when you exercise you need to sweat, to get the maximum benefit, and that will be harder the older you get.'

I struggled at the start. It felt effortful, and I had to dig deep to see it through. I started by warming up on a cross-trainer for six minutes before moving to the rowing machine for five minutes. The stepper followed – one step at a time initially, then a double step. I always tried to complete the eight minutes by not holding on to the bars at the side but that was easier said than done. By this point I was usually sweating. Next came the climber where I completed one minute gently and then one minute at full tilt. The aerobic section ended on the flex-trainer, which is like a cross trainer but more dynamic. You could take longer strides, and it was great for stretching my arms and shoulders. It was possible to follow a virtual route from the coast of New Zealand's South Island to the wonders of the Yosemite National Park in California. Before leaving I headed upstairs to complete my strength and balance training.

Developing an exercise routine is not easy: it takes three weeks to start to form a habit and three months to make it a lifestyle choice. This is even more challenging for people with Parkinson's due to apathy and other barriers to motivation such as fatigue, depression and anxiety, but over the next few weeks the routine began to feel easier, and I started to enjoy it more. I felt fitter, stronger, and was able to concentrate better in work.

The routine I developed didn't just involve the machines. I would get up, shave and take my medications at 6.00 am; I found that setting a reminder helped so I packed and set out my gym bag the night before I was due to go. Breakfast of overnight oats was prepared and set ready to grab quickly from the fridge on my way out the door. The drive lasted fifteen minutes, always to the same music, and after parking my car I made a beeline for locker twenty-three every morning. It's the unspoken rule among the early morning members to use the same locker every time – it is the small things like this which minimises the effort particularly first thing in the morning.

I had a review meeting with Mark every three months when he would gradually increase the resistance to improve my fitness level. It truly was a personalised plan. What Mark was able to do was to set regular goals that I could achieve and that was the key. They were achievable. There is nothing worse than starting out on a course of action only to realise that you are not going to achieve it despite your best efforts as the bar has been set too high too quickly.

There were differences between when I had exercised before and how I was exercising now. Firstly, I was on my own, isolated and not part of a team, so if I didn't turn up no one chased me. Secondly, I was forty-one and not seventeen anymore so I had to respect that my body was older. Finally, I couldn't ignore that I was now living with Parkinson's. In addition to the gym I started exercising with a friend as this introduced a degree of accountability. If I didn't turn up he was going to chase it up and I would need a good excuse. It's also easier to push your own limits when you exercise with someone else as it harnesses the power of competition.

One day my friend Jules, who was a keen road cyclist, enquired whether I had a bike. I replied that I didn't but described how I always enjoyed cycling in the gym.

'I'll take you out. There is nothing quite like being in the fresh air,' he added.

That was the start of my love for cycling. He brought around his spare racing bike and adjusted the height of the seat. I had already been down to my local bike shop and bought a white helmet (a strong one!), a cycling top, padded leggings and a pair of cleats. I was trying to make myself more like Davis Phinney, the American cyclist, and less like a 'MAMIL' (middle-aged man in Lycra.)

We met every Sunday morning at 7.30 am, one week at my house and the next at his. He pre-planned the route including the distance and the height that we would climb. The roads were always clear at that time on a Sunday morning. I felt free and alive. There is no better feeling after gritting your teeth and digging deep than reaching the top of a hill. One Sunday I was struggling up an especially steep incline when Jules shouted at me in encouragement.

'I think I am going to have to stop,' I panted. But I persevered and eventually reached the top to be greeted with the most beautiful sunrise. The rays of light pierced the dawn fog as the sheep grazed happily in the field below us. Jules was right – there is something special about exercising in the fresh air. At the end of each ride there is a slow incline uphill from the village church to our house. Every time I passed the church Jules would shout, 'Are you ready?' He would encourage me to keep turning those pedals as quickly and efficiently as I could. The challenge segment began to record on Strava, and I could compare how long it took each ride. Some days I had plenty in the tank, other days I couldn't maintain my speed and had to slow down.

It had taken me two years to get on a road bike post-diagnosis and I was thoroughly enjoying it. It was very social, and by the end of Sunday I was already forty percent of the way to my target of two and a half hours of high intensity exercise for the week.

After we had been cycling for about six months, I came across an advertisement from Parkinson's UK who were running an event called Pedal for Parkinson's. There were various locations across the UK but the closest was Stratford-Upon-Avon. You could choose to complete twenty, fifty or a hundred miles. We had a discussion and decided we would settle for the twenty miles. That may not seem like far but to me it was. We trained hard, slowly building the length of our Sunday morning excursions to ten miles, then twelve, then fourteen, then sixteen and finally eighteen, all with different degrees of climbing. We were leaving the twenty miles to the actual event.

The day of the event dawned, and Jules arrived early. As we set off, the morning dew reflected the sun, creating a carpet of diamonds. The air was already warming, and we knew it was going to be a hot one. We waited to be called for our slot and when the hooter sounded, we set off in tandem. We travelled through villages, up country roads, most of it very picturesque. There was a welcome water stop at the ten-mile mark before we completed the rest of the ride in around eighty minutes. I had a great sense of achievement that day, I felt proud of what we had done, and it was a very positive experience overall.

In April 2018, two years after I had been diagnosed, I heard a knock at the door and upon opening it discovered a brand-new black Pinnacle racing bike gleaming in the warm afternoon sun. I looked up and down our park to determine who may have left but the park was empty. Suddenly, my eye was drawn to a piece of paper that had been attached to the frame of the bike. I took it off carefully and unfolded it to find a handwritten message, which simply said,

> Jonny, please accept this bike from me as I know how important exercise is for those with Parkinson's and how much you enjoy cycling. The bike is brand new, fully paid for, and there is no option for you not to accept it!! Just enjoy the cycling with family and friends and know that it is given with much love and affection.
> A friend.

I found out six months later that Jules had put the bike outside my house. I am forever grateful to him for his support and encouragement, particularly in those early stages after diagnosis. His contribution was vital in helping me to establish good exercise routines and pushing my limits to maximise my function. Thanks to Mark and his contribution I regained fitness levels I believed I had long lost.

When we consider what can be done to help those with Parkinson's to adapt there is a lot of focus on the role of the healthcare community, government and charities, but it is important not to overlook the impact of an individual. Time, care, encouragement and generosity all have enormous potential to help people adapt to change and none of these require training, education or expertise, just humanity.

CHAPTER 4

Muscle Memory

One morning, a few months after I started going to the gym, I was tidying the garage when I stumbled upon my old jump rope gathering dust. It was at least five years since it had last been used and given my diagnosis, now looked more like a risk for falling than a helpful piece of fitness equipment. Deciding my days of skipping were behind me, I removed it from the shelf and tossed it into the pile destined for the tip. However, a few hours later I returned to the garage, recovered the rope and placed it back where I had found it. Something had bothered me about throwing it away. At first, I couldn't put my finger on what it was, but later I realised throwing it away would have meant conceding a loss to Parkinson's. I was assuming my limitations rather than testing them.

When I discovered I had a progressive condition with no treatment or ability to prevent further damage it felt a little bit like being strapped into a harness on a roller coaster and sent on my way, in a manner that wasn't fun but terrifying. The course was set and I had no control over it; no capacity to slow, stop or change.

Without realising it, I had fallen into a pattern of deterministic thinking believing that the outcomes of my Parkinson's were fixed and unalterable. However, whilst we know that progression will inevitably take place over time, so much else is unclear. Both the rate and pattern of progress are unknown and there is huge variability from one person to the next. Science has not exhausted all the possibilities but is constantly advancing and is exploring how we can modify the course by exercise and non-pharmaceutical interventions like diet. Finally, and perhaps more importantly, quality of life outcomes are not dependant solely on pathology. As health professionals we sometimes forget that there is more to our function and quality of life than the sum of our biology. We have psychological, social and spiritual dimensions which impact in ways we can't always measure. They are important in motivation, endurance, resilience and courage, and the positive news is that they are much less fixed and open to modification. There may not yet be a cure for Parkinson's, but we can reframe our thinking, we can seek out new social interactions and change aspects of our environment. As we considered earlier, we are not left without choices. Where healthcare professionals, care circles and society in general can help is in supporting those living with PD to make positive ones.

Finding the rope piqued my curiosity and posed a challenge, so it wasn't long before I found myself reaching up, once more, to remove it from the shelf. I brought it outside onto the driveway and unzipped the cover.

DOI: 10.1201/9781003600671-4

The rope was neatly wound up and secured by two Velcro straps. Cylindrical weights like those found on a wind chime were stacked underneath. Slotting one into each of the handles I lifted the rope out. It felt familiar and comfortable in my grasp. I held my two arms straight in front of me and pulled on the rope until I could feel it taut against the back of my ankles before releasing the tension just enough to enable the rope to touch the ground. A small knot formed in my stomach that was a mixture of nerves and excitement. With limited movement in one wrist would I really be able to manage this? I did not want to have to explain to Heather I had tripped whilst skipping!

Inhaling deeply, I pulled the rope over my head and jumped. It felt oddly easy. I repeated the same movement faster and faster quickly finding rhythm. The rope hit the ground at the same time interval each rotation – a steady, constant whoosh. I was so happy to be skipping again that at first I didn't notice my left arm was moving normally. Not only had my range of movement improved but the left wrist was rotating at speed and keeping up with the right one. All evidence of asymmetry had vanished. It was an unbelievable feeling and I was stunned. When I stopped skipping and attempted to rotate my wrist the signs of Parkinson's returned, but when I restarted they disappeared again.

I was to discover after research that this is a common phenomenon. This is muscle memory in action. Activities which are learnt and repeatedly rehearsed to become instinctive are programmed in different motor pathways in the brain. In this case skipping was able to access movement in my wrist in a way I couldn't do otherwise. I was so excited. It felt as though the horizon of my world had suddenly expanded. If this were true for skipping then what else would I discover?

There are many personal stories where those with significant motor symptoms and loss of function can experience noticeable improvement when they dance, play table tennis or play a musical instrument. Sometimes individuals stop a hobby because of frustration that they cannot undertake it to a previous standard or level. It is not easy to continue, for example painting, when you have stiffness or a tremor. We are usually our own worst critics, and no one relishes functioning below par. The truth is that I was not skipping as long, quickly or accurately as I would have before, but the point is, I was moving my wrist and that was helping my joint and muscles and more importantly countering the stiffness and rigidity that Parkinson's was causing. Muscle memory will exist for anything we have repeatedly rehearsed or practised, and former hobbies or activities may be the easiest place to start. But even after a diagnosis taking up a new hobby will help to develop new muscle memory which may prove beneficial later.

The muscle memory when using a jump rope was created twenty-five years before I was diagnosed with Parkinson's when I had attended an American high school at the age of sixteen. This was to prove a formative year.

––––––––––––––

Gordon Graham was a very successful lawyer in Boston, Massachusetts, who, after being involved in a near-fatal car accident, was awarded substantial damages. Graham used the compensation to set up a scholarship programme in honour of his parents who were born and raised in Ireland. The programme funded a secondary school student from County Down or County Mayo, the counties from which they originated, on alternate years. The scholarship aimed to allow a student the opportunity to experience living with an American host family and attend an American high school in Clinton, a small town, about one hour west of Boston.

In 1990 it was County Down's turn, and our headteacher announced this once-in-a-lifetime opportunity, during a school assembly, inviting anyone who was completing their GCSE examinations that summer to apply. The successful candidate across all the schools would be decided by an essay entitled 'Why should you be awarded the scholarship this year?'

That evening I told my parents I was interested in applying. A student from my school had previously won the scholarship, so Mum helpfully arranged to speak with him and his family. As I listened intently to his experiences, I realised this was a unique opportunity for adventure that would never arise again. It would afford me the chance to travel, explore and play different sports. I lifted my pen and started to write the essay. I had decided it was too good an opportunity to miss.

A few months later I arrived home from school to discover a letter on the hall carpet. I could immediately recognise from the stamps and the postage mark it had been posted from Boston and at once a mixture of pure excitement and nausea bubbled. Opening the letter I saw that it had been sent from the law offices of Gordon Graham, and the butterflies in my stomach went into overdrive. The letter continued, informing me that I would be staying with a host family called the DiTullios. Claudio and Kathy had three children, Kristen who was seventeen, Adrianna who was thirteen and Jeremy who was seven.

I had indicated on my application form that I wanted to play American football for Clinton High School. (The rules in the USA are strict when a student from outside the country arrives on a scholarship program.) You cannot participate in a sport in the American school if you have represented your home school in that same sport. I qualified to play either American football or soccer, as it was called in the US, as I had played rugby at school. Training for American football started the second week of August and attendance was compulsory to have any chance of making the team, so my flight had been booked for the first Saturday in August.

On the 4 August 1991 I found myself peering through the window of a plane watching as it descended over the Boston skyline. I had no idea what would lie ahead. Collecting my bags from the carousel I put on a neon orange baseball cap emblazoned with the word 'Clinton.' The DiTullios had posted it to Northern Ireland and told me to wear it in the arrivals lounge so they could identify me.

I walked through the arrivals hall and past sign after sign with people's names and taxi companies eagle-eyed to find their fare. I had taken the cap off as I was feeling very self-conscious and just held it in my hand. I never really suited baseball caps. Claudio was to tell me later in the year that when they saw me walking with the orange cap, they had to take a double look at this five-foot-eight-inch, thin-as-a-rake child from Northern Ireland. I am not sure what Gordon Graham had relayed to them, but they were expecting to see a six-foot-one-inch, two-hundred-and-fifteen-pound teenager, built like a tank with muscles to burn. They envisaged a linebacker who would be a great addition as a defensive team member of the Clinton High School American football team. I was introduced to all their family, including their nephew David who was the high school football captain for the coming year. He had a very firm handshake and he *was* six-foot-one and two hundred and fifteen pounds!

'Have you thought what position you might play?' they asked on the hour-long journey back to Clinton. 'It is a very physical game and we don't want you to get injured,' they added with a concerned tone. I was a big National Football League (NFL) fan and usually watched the highlights show on Channel Four on a Sunday evening. The position I most enjoyed watching was the kicker, who is a strategic and integral part of the game. There were two kickers that I followed – Matt Bahr of the New York Giants and Morten Andersen of the New Orleans Saints. Andersen was a barefooted kicker who reportedly had his left foot insured for over a million dollars. He rarely missed and in 1990 Barr kicked the winning field goal in the last second of the NFC Championship Game to take the New York Giants to the Superbowl. 'I think I will try out to be the kicker,' I said. They were a little taken aback. 'High school kids can throw and run with the ball, but we have never had anyone who can actually kick it,' they added.

I spent the day unpacking but after tea it was suggested we head to the local school pitch as everyone was interested to see whether I could kick an American football. Claudio brought his brother-in-law along who was an American football referee, and whose nickname was 'Goose,' (I never found out why he had that name). Despite jet lag I spent two hours kicking ball after ball. I kicked off from a tee, practised kicking extra points and longer field goals. After we finally called it a day, and unbeknown to me, 'Goose' phoned the head coach of the Clinton High School American football team and told him he had found him a kid who could kick.

The following day began the week of the captain's practice where we would train for three hours every day. One hour of general fitness, one hour of practising pre-planned plays and one hour in the gym lifting weights. I have never been as tired as I was that Friday night. And that was just week one.

The following Monday morning was the start of coach's week where there was training in the morning and afternoon, and if they didn't think enough effort was being put in, you were also brought back for an evening session. This week we had to wear full kit. The sun was splitting the skies, beaming onto our metal helmets, and I felt like Robocop.

Archie Cataldi was a well-respected, no-nonsense, old-school head coach who had decades of experience and had been putting teams through their paces for years, but he had never coached a kicker before. 'So, you think you can kick, kid?' – peering at me sceptically over his glasses. 'He's got the luck of the Irish,' Dave answered in my support. Dave was the special team's coach and oversaw set plays and my specific training regime, but it was Cataldi who would decide when I was to be used in the game. He was the strategic mastermind. 'Let's see!' he said.

Every day we were weighed at the start and the end of each session, to ensure we had drunk enough water in between. That was the first time I learned to link the benefits of physical activity and hydration for your brain and body and is a lesson I have never forgotten. After stretching to warm up, Cataldi would roar and make us run ten times around the pitch. It was tough in the heat. They didn't have water bottles, they had water barrels, about fifteen in total all lined up on a table, where you could grab a cup after every lap that you completed. At the end, we guzzled the water down, took our helmets off and poured it on our heads to cool down. Next, we went through the playbook; multiple predetermined plays where each player had a specific task to learn.

At the end of the morning session, I had the opportunity to demonstrate what I had learnt, but I was nervous as I had never kicked in full gridiron. As a snap came back, Kevin, the holder, whose nickname was 'Geek,' caught it and placed it on the tee. I drilled it high and as straight as an arrow through the posts. '2.1 seconds,' Dave shouted. I had no idea I was being timed by a stopwatch. 'Again!' Cataldi shouted. I drilled another this time in '1.8 seconds.' 'The kid *can* kick,' Cataldi said beaming from ear to ear, 'but can he do it under pressure in a game?'

Afternoon sessions were less about cardio fitness with more emphasis on weights and lots of practice. Dave had produced a personalised training regime especially for me which included thirty minutes of skipping with a jump rope and a specific leg weight program. 'You don't need arm muscles to burn. You just need the legs,' he said. Over the next weeks and months, I became adept at skipping, being able to add in a double jump and crossing over jumps. I felt like a boxer, developing my own rhythm.

On the Wednesday of that week Cataldi wanted to see if I could punt. A punt is when the ball is snapped back directly into the hands of a player who kicks it aiming to get the ball to go as long and as high as he can. A good punt has a long hang time giving your team the chance to tackle the opposition player as close to their end zone as possible, putting pressure on the offence to make a mistake and hence gain good field position. The average hang time for a punt in the NFL is 4.3 to 5.0 seconds with an average distance of forty-two yards. Dave set everything up and when the snap came back directly to me, I caught the ball, took a step forward, kicked and sent it flying through the air spiralling like a torpedo. The training pitch was behind the high school and there was a row of businesses that ran along one side of it with a high fence. As I watched, the ball cleared the fence and struck the tarmac making the almightiest bang. All the other players stopped and looked up. 'Did he just kick that into the car park?' someone said. 'He sure did,' Cataldi said laughing. The hang time was 3.9 seconds.

We trained every day after school. Games were played on Friday night, under floodlights, in front of a crowd of three thousand locals. High school football is a big deal in the USA. We didn't wear normal clothes to high school on a game day. Instead, everyone on the team was allowed to wear their game shirt – I was number thirty-eight. Our school lockers were decorated, wishing us all the best, and the cheerleaders spent lunch working on the final changes to their routines. It was just like the movies. On the evening of the first game of the season we all met in the school gym beforehand to travel to the match together. Cataldi gave a rousing team talk and I felt the hairs rise on the back of my neck as everyone stood to applause. Arriving at the ground I spotted a large sign saying, 'Welcome to Fuller Field, the home of the Clinton Gaels.' We were called the Gaels as a nod to the rich Irish heritage in Clinton. We had a half man–half horse mystical figure on the side of our helmets, except these Gaels were carrying a football under their arms. Music was playing, loudly, and there was a PA announcer, popcorn and stands selling team merchandise. This was high stakes football.

We were playing a team from a division above us in the first game. The first three quarters were a tight affair.

There were just minutes left on the clock at the end of the game when Dave told me to warm up. Our quarterback, Greg, threw a pinpoint accurate pass. We were 4th down and 3, just fifteen yards from their end zone. I looked at Dave expectantly, poised, ready to run onto the pitch to kick a field goal and seal the win when I heard Cataldi's booming voice behind me. 'Not tonight, kid,' he said. As I had missed an extra point kick earlier in the game, he did not want to take the risk and indicated the play that he wanted instead.

The snap went smoothly. Greg faked to go to the right spun around and handed the ball off to our running back. A huge hole appeared in their defensive line and the three-thousand-strong crowd was whipped up into a frenzy as he dived into the end zone. It was twelve points to six. The referee blew his whistle. We had won. After the game Dave came to me in the changing room and reassured me that my time would come. I realised that night I needed to be as mentally strong and fit as I was physically.

On Monday morning the local paper, the *Clinton Daily Item*, had a full-page spread summarising the game on the previous Friday. I bought two copies, one for me to keep and one to post home to keep my family up to date with what had happened. I did this after every game. Little did I know that my mum was sticking them all into a scrapbook to record the events that unfolded.

We played twelve games in total that season, always on a Friday, six at home and six away. Kevin and I were a well-oiled machine by the end of the season. I knocked over extra point after extra point, kicked off well and continued to get good distance and hang time on my punts. As the season progressed my leg muscles became stronger, my hamstrings loosened and my technique developed. My form was consistent and Cataldi increasingly used me in game play. Punting became a strength and I was so pleased to read a quote in one match report from Coach Cataldi in the *Clinton Daily Item* describing it as 'a real jewel.' In the following game I ran onto the pitch to punt. The snap was good and I laced the ball. I had never made such a good contact before and watched as the ball flew through the air with the floodlights glistening. It travelled sixty-seven yards. Dave ripped his headset off and punched the air. It was beautiful to watch, and it was a Clinton American football school record that stood for many years.

In the final game I was given the chance to come on and attempt my first field goal of the season. Kevin knelt into position just like he had done on numerous occasions, except this kick was further away from the posts. 'This is it,' he said, 'this is your moment.' 'This is our moment,' I replied. I couldn't have done it without him or indeed the whole team. It was so cold both of us were wearing gloves and you could see our breath in the icy evening air. I took my customary two steps back and then two steps to the right from the tee and slowed my breathing. 'Don't drop it,' I said to Kevin. 'Don't miss it,' he replied. We were set, I took a deep breath, exhaled, put my head down and followed through to the target. The next day as I read the final game report I smiled. 'Acheson set up for a thirty-two-yard field goal. The Gaels kicker booted the ball straight through the uprights to give Clinton a 10–0 lead. In the last game I had finally added that elusive field goal to my achievements. My statistics for the season were 18 out of 21 extra points and one field goal. An unexpected but welcome bonus was that I was named as the Midland-Wachusett Division C all-star team kicker.

On the Wednesday after the final game Cataldi called me into his office. 'I have never coached a kicker before,' he said. 'I was hesitant, but you have proved yourself and you should be very proud.' I had won his confidence but far more important was the impact it had on my own. Throughout the season I learned how to overcome disappointment, turn a negative into a positive and convince people that a course of action was the right one. Just because you haven't tried something before isn't a reason that you shouldn't.

Memory not only exists for rehearsed repetitive activities but also exists for emotions. Everyone can recount sounds or smells which immediately evoke feelings of pleasure, comfort or fear. There is a certain smell of coconut oil that at once transports me to holidays on the beach, whereas the smell of pineapple more than thirty years later still evokes the fear of being caught in a force 8 gale on the Lord Rank tall ship. We also develop memory in the realm of thinking, establishing core beliefs in childhood which subconsciously influence us as adults. Some of these core beliefs are adaptive and aid us in the process of change. Others are less so and can unknowingly impede us. Developing greater awareness of such core beliefs can be helpful in identifying areas where our thinking can be modified to become more adaptive. An individual's psychology has important implications for their management and so it is important to try and understand it. Equally, having knowledge of significant life events can be pivotal. They can be employed in management by engaging memory in a positive way. The year I spent in America is one such example. This opportunity was, in one regard, a huge adventure, but in another regard a time of isolation and duress. I found myself alone at sixteen years old in a country in which I previously knew no one having to very quickly adapt to a different culture. I was immensely fortunate in being attached to the DiTullios who were so welcoming and became my surrogate family, but it still took time to develop these relationships. The comfort and security of home and mum were thousands of miles away in Northern Ireland, and these were days long before the invention of the internet and mobile phones when communication with home was largely by the slow process of post. I had to learn to contain my own anxiety, to take responsibility for my own decisions and become independent. I made mistakes, there were tears and occasional days when I wondered why I had ever written the letter, but I survived and as the year progressed, increasingly thrived. In April 1992 I decided to take the bus on my own from Boston to Orlando because I wanted to visit Walt Disney World. Thirty-two hours and 1325 miles later after multiple changes, including a 4 am cheeseburger and some iced tea, I finally arrived. What this year taught me above all was that pressure hadn't crushed me, that I could withstand more than I thought. It taught me resilience and every gram developed has proved in life to be far more precious than gold. When I have faced subsequent pressure and adversity, I have been able to use the memories from this year to fortify my resolve, encourage endurance and sustain hope.

CHAPTER 5

Learning

Change as we have considered is a constant of life. No matter how hard we try it is impossible to shield ourselves from it. But how we respond to change is not fixed. One of my favourite programmes as a child was a cartoon called Mr Ben. Each episode would begin with Mr Ben attired in a work suit and bowler hat entering a shop whereupon he would change outfits before embarking on a related adventure. Like Mr Ben adaptability can wear many guises. Rather than considering it a single attribute, it is perhaps more helpful to view adaptability as a paint box with a variety of colours for different situations. The skill is blending the right colours and understanding their individual contribution to the overall picture. However, a paint box on its own is insufficient; tools are needed to apply them to a canvas. Allied to the ability to adapt are the skills essential for learning.

Working as an Emergency Medicine consultant, even in good health, is both physically and emotionally taxing, so it is not unusual to develop other specialist interests to make the job more sustainable. Shortly after I was appointed as a consultant in Leicester, I was offered the opportunity to participate in undergraduate education. I did not hesitate. Medical students from the University of Leicester rotate through our department every seven weeks and I took over the role of organising and supervising this block of their education.

As a medical student I hadn't always enjoyed the process of learning. Teaching ward rounds were frequently intimidating experiences. Akin to ducklings who follow their mother, a line of six or so students, in oversized white coats, would follow the consultant as they reviewed their patients on their round. We would stand anxiously around the patient's bedside, hoping we would know the answer to whatever question was about to be asked and desperate to avoid the cutting remarks that would follow if we didn't. Frequently the question asked was so difficult there was not a chance anyone would know the answer. And that was the point. Its purpose was to reveal how little we knew. It was learning by humiliation and fear.

But when I started my first training job in Emergency Medicine, I encountered a different learning experience. Mr Fee, the Head of Service and my supervising consultant, was a natural educator whose teaching stemmed from a love of what he did and a desire to help everyone realise their full potential. Patient, good-natured and humble, he considered every case a learning opportunity. I recall a shift, shortly after I had started my placement, when a patient presented to minors having fallen and hit

 DOI: 10.1201/9781003600671-5

her forehead on the pavement. She had a wide, gaping wound that spanned her whole forehead. Even with my limited experience I knew it could not be fixed by a normal stitch. 'I will show you how to close that,' Mr. Fee had offered when I had asked for help. He pulled across a stool, sat on one side of the patient, and after the local anaesthetic had taken effect, he diligently began to insert absorbable stitches into the layer of tissue below the skin, teaching me as he did so. After he had inserted them all, he started to tie each of them individually, starting from the middle and working towards each opposite end. Once completed, we started with the outer layer of skin, he worked so quickly he covered sixty percentage of the length of the wound by the time I had inserted four stitches. He looked up with a reassuring smile, removed his glasses and gloves and said, 'You are doing a great job. You can finish up. Make sure you come into cubicle seven when you have finished.' I was a little apprehensive but I completed the task and tidied away all the equipment. When I walked into cubicle seven, Mr. Fee beckoned for me to sit down. 'Tea or coffee?' he asked and proceeded with his debrief.

Mr Fee demonstrated that the key to good education is to engage, enthuse and encourage your audience. He also showed how education can impact patients, staff and service provision and at an early stage of postgraduate training instilled my own desire to become involved and to help others learn. Many have encouraged me along the way, but he was the ignition for my medical education journey, and when I teach today, I hope it's the Mr Fee way.

As a student I presupposed that learning was mostly knowledge acquisition. The more you knew and the quicker you knew it, the better you would become. However, as I progressed through training, I began to realise that there are certain attributes as important as intellect, and prior to developing my role as an educator, I first had to develop as a learner.

To learn requires humility because learning involves failing. Anyone who has ever watched an infant trying to take their first steps knows this. No one sets out to fail but there must be a willingness to accept it as a possibility and this depends on acknowledging that we are not perfect but fallible. If we are governed by a fear of failure and do everything to avoid it, our development will be hindered, and we will stagnate. We often learn far more from one mistake than a hundred successes, but it requires a second quality – resolution – to help us overcome the fear to try in the first place or to get 'back on the horse' after failing.

Throughout the year we review over two hundred thousand cases in our ED. Most are treated successfully and with good outcome. However, we cannot escape our humanity, and mistakes happen despite every best effort. Though rare in relation to the many correct decisions, those that do occur are impactful and can become permanently seared into your memory: the margins for error in the ED are small and the consequences significant. Despite happening more than twenty years ago I still vividly recall a harrowing experience with a slit lamp. This is a piece of equipment employed when you are attempting to remove a foreign body from an eye using a fine needle. Looking into the slit lamp helps magnify everything and makes the process easier.

It was an afternoon shift, and a welder had presented with a foreign body in his eye. I applied some local anaesthetic eye drops to numb his eye and brought him to the cubicle with the slit lamp where I instructed him to put his chin on the chin rest and correctly positioned him so that his forehead rested on a plastic white bar that transected the lamp. I explained what I was going to do and how important it was that he keep his head still. He was nervous, so much so that I could see that he was sweating. As I pulled my chair in towards the slit lamp and brought the needle into view, I slowly moved it towards the eye so that I could flick the piece of metal out when the needle reached the eyeball. But as I was doing so, unbeknown to me, the patient had taken his forehead off the plastic bar and moved it backwards ever so slightly. I was nervous myself and because I was so focused on what I was doing I had missed his movement. When I touched his eye with the needle he panicked and, in the process, jolted his head forward until it hit the plastic bar he should have been resting on. The forward momentum caused the needle to lodge in his eye: I reeled backwards, aghast at what had just happened. He reeled backwards, scrunched his eyes and as he did so, I noticed that he was starting to cry blood. That was it, I thought, my Emergency Medicine career was over before it had started.

It transpired that I had made a superficial nick in the white of his eye and it healed quickly and without any long-term harm. However, incidents like this leave imprints and take time to process. You return home at the end of the shift and it is hard to switch off. When your confidence has been knocked the instinct is to become over-cautious, further diminishing confidence and feeding a negative spiral. Yet, returning to work on your next shift, you must be ready for all possible scenarios. A critically injured child or a patient in cardiac arrest will need a calm doctor with a clear mind. Reflection is essential to improve and avoid repeating the same mistakes, but it is a skill ED doctors must learn to do quickly. There is not time for significant introspection or to consider how we might be feeling; we must be adept at compartmentalising and processing emotions and resolute to arrive focused and composed at the start of the next shift.

Learning continues until the day you hang up your stethoscope. As a medical student and doctor in training, you learn a small amount of detail about a lot of conditions. However, as you increasingly specialise this is replaced by deeper knowledge of fewer conditions, those relevant to cases that you are seeing day to day in your job. In addition to humility and resolution, good learners need curiosity. They ask the question 'Why?' Early in training this natural curiosity results in a rapid expansion of knowledge. However, as a consultant the focus is gradually directed away from passing exams towards improving patient care, gaining practical experience and improving the systems we work in. It begins to extend to questioning conventions and protocols, asking, why do we do things the way we do? Such questions inevitably start a quest for answers. Sometimes they can be found in medical literature but when they can't or when the search raises further questions the seed is sown for research.

Education and research are two sides of the learning coin. Research helps us learn and learning helps us educate. Education teaches the practice which research establishes and so all good educators, must to some degree, also be researchers.

Toddlers frequently present to the ED for the removal of objects which have become stuck in their nostrils. All manner of things can be inserted from beads to Lego to rolled-up pieces of paper. When I started working in Northern Ireland all these cases were referred to the ear, nose and throat (ENT) doctors who removed the item using various instruments. If that failed, then they needed to go to theatre to have it removed under general anaesthetic. I had read in the medical literature about a different method that was called 'the kissing technique.' It required the parent to sit on a chair cradling their child in their arms. They would then tilt them backwards slightly compressing the nostril that didn't have the foreign body. After inhaling they would place their lips around their child's mouth, as if kissing them. Finally, when they had formed a tight seal, they blew a short, sharp, burst of air into the child's mouth. The mouth or the oral cavity is connected to the nasal cavity so when the air is blown in at speed it creates enough force to go up the nose, into the nasal cavity, and displace the object. That's why the parent needed to compress the opposite nostril. If they didn't, the force would not be strong enough to cause displacement. All sorts flew out with breakneck speed, sometimes bouncing off the floor.

Over a fifteen-month period we followed one hundred and sixteen cases and found that the success rate of the technique was 48.8% with a lower rate of instrumentation and general anaesthetic. Following publication of this work the kissing technique became standard practice in our ED and in other EDs across the world.

Learning is an integral part of adaption. Parkinson's changes the daily landscape of our lives. What was familiar is gradually transformed. There is a new language. Words like dyskinesia, bradykinesia, agonist and deep brain stimulation become part of your vocabulary, and even familiar words like freezing and 'off' take on a new meaning. You must learn new rhythms and routines to incorporate medication schedules, exercise and vocal training and there are new experiences to be understood such as anxiety and sleep disorder. There is so much to learn, especially in the beginning, that it often feels overwhelming. I encountered this even though my medical training should have provided a better basis than most from which to start. Familiarity wraps itself like a cosy blanket around all of us. It is uncomfortable to move from under it and the temptation is to remain where we are. It is not only difficult, but it can also be frightening because learning anew introduces the possibility of getting things wrong. It requires accepting we need help at a point in life where we have become more accustomed to providing it than asking for it. In this regard to navigate we must become students and employ the same characteristics of resolution humility and curiosity. When we encounter something, we don't understand we have to be willing to ask those who do, to be curious and to seek answers to the question why. There may not always be an answer but perhaps in asking it we will trigger that curiosity in someone else that will lead to research and find the answer in the future. And as healthcare professionals we must do the same: remain humble, listening and learning from those living with the condition and not permitting the pressures of time and resources to extinguish curiosity. We must be willing to try things to see if they work and not give up if they don't but remain resolute in moving forwards, and herein lies a final essential attribute in learning – perseverance.

CHAPTER 6

Perseverance

If curiosity and resolution oil the wheel of learning, it is perseverance that keeps it turning. Although I work as a consultant in the Emergency Department that was not always the plan.

Returning from America in 1992 I began studying A-levels, with the clear goal of pursuing a career in medicine, and was fortunate to eventually secure a place to study at Queen's University Belfast (QUB). Not only did I study at Queen's it was also where I met my wife, Heather. The weekend before I was due to start medical school, I had signed up for a Freshers event at an ice rink. During the evening a friend in second year pointed me in the direction of three people who were on my course. Although I can't recall exactly what I said, I can remember that one of the three was very easy to talk too. She had the brownest of eyes, her hair was in a neat bob and she was wearing a light blue checked shirt and a pair of black leggings. I am not sure what her initial impression was of me as I had on a pair of ripped jeans, a crinkled t-shirt and a mop of curly hair which I had stopped brushing when I was fifteen, but it was evidently not too bad. A few months later we began dating and after much hard work, countless exams and a lot of fun we graduated, started work and married in 2000.

When I had first applied to study medicine I envisioned working as a rural GP in Northern Ireland and for the duration of undergraduate training these plans did not change. Rotations provided experience across many different hospital specialities, but nothing competed with the appeal of working in the local community. I liked the prospect of continuity of patient care, looking after all the family whatever illness or pathology presented. Following graduation and having completed a year of core training I had several options available to train as a GP. At that time the most common routes were to apply to the specialist three-year training programme for general practice or to complete a two-year programme in an acute hospital followed by a year of training in a GP surgery. However, these were highly competitive programmes and despite several interviews I found myself missing out each time. After hours of study, multiple examinations and six years of hard work this was a discouraging and frustrating time. There was an inevitable impact on my confidence and moments of significant self-doubt. Why was I failing? What did I need to change to bring about a different outcome? Looking back, this was also a time with lots of questions which had no clear answers. Many days felt difficult, and it was sometimes a battle to keep pressing forward but my faith, that my worth is not found in the sum of my successes and failures, helped me to keep persevering and in the end, I decided to opt for the less secure pathway of making up my own rotation and submitted an application for an Emergency Medicine job in the hospital in which I was working at the time. Like general practice, this job would provide opportunity to practice the breadth of medicine across the range of age groups and I knew it would prove to be a valuable experience. It was based in a district general hospital in Northern Ireland.

On my first night shift in the ED, I was the only doctor working in the department after two o'clock in the morning as beyond this time senior cover was provided by the on-call consultant from home. This would not happen today, but back then it was normal. It was learning by being thrown in at the deep end and it was terrifying. I was responsible for seeing every patient that came through the doors regardless of their presentation, which could range from a minor laceration sustained on a sports field to a major trauma from a road traffic accident, and I did not want to have to repeatedly wake the consultant on call without good reason.

At 02.35 the red phone rang. I liken this to the bat phone. It indicated a serious situation was about to unfold and that the patient arriving was critically ill. The ED nurse wrote down a summary of the case from ambulance control and then verbalised what she had written. 'Red call, five minutes,' she said, 'forty-five-year old male with sudden shortness of breath and chest pain.' There was an immediate surge of adrenaline.

When the patient arrived, he looked pale in the manner that suggested serious illness. He was very short of breath and unable to speak in full sentences and I noticed that he had a plaster of Paris cast on his lower left leg. Reaching a diagnosis in medicine is a methodical process. We are trained to use answers from a series of specific questions that form the patient's history and objective observations from our clinical examination, to construct a management plan and determine appropriate investigations and treatment. When you are a medical student, this process is not time critical. It is possible to be thorough and methodically free from any significant constraint. But this was a different matter; now the pressure was intense.

I began to follow the frameworks as I had been taught. I asked if his shortness of breath had come on suddenly – he nodded. Was it sharp – he nodded. Was it worse when he tried to breathe in – he nodded. As the nurse attached the monitors, I observed his heart rate was high, his breathing rate was fast and he was not getting sufficient oxygen to his blood despite being attached to a high-flow mask. His condition was deteriorating rapidly. Very quickly I assessed that I didn't have the luxury of following my well-practised history taking. Time mattered. Judgment was necessary to understand the most salient information. I needed to adapt.

I suspected a deep vein thrombosis or clot had likely formed in the lower leg with the cast on it. Part of it had possibly dislodged, travelling through the heart before becoming stuck in one of the lungs' main blood vessels, blocking the blood supply and preventing gas exchange in the lungs. If this wasn't reversed the body would run out of oxygen and the patient would go into cardiac arrest. I fast bleeped the medical registrar, the most experienced doctor in the hospital after midnight, through the hospital communication system. His pager would alert him to attend the resuscitation room (resus) ASAP. However, the length of time it would take for him to arrive would depend on whether he was tied up in another critical situation. I started inserting a large cannula into the patient's arm and took some blood. I knew he needed a clot-busting medication as his blood pressure reading indicated his condition was life threatening, but this required a senior decision – there was only so much I could do on my own. Every minute felt like thirty until the medical registrar finally arrived. He calmly explained to the nurses what he needed and discussed with the patient what he was going to do. As the medication was being given, I watched in relief as his heart rate decreased, his breathing rate decreased, his oxygen levels rose and his blood pressure increased.

This is the routine and daily experience of work in resus and it is often every bit as dramatic as portrayed on television. I never have forgotten the first time I successfully shocked a patient in cardiac arrest with a defibrillator or relocated a joint. I had intended to apply for a different specialty at the end of the six months but within two months I was hooked and decided to remain in the ED.

After changing course from general practice to undertake Emergency Medicine training, the next step was to pass postgraduate examinations and apply to the Northern Ireland Emergency Medicine higher specialist training program. The day you graduate is only the beginning of the learning journey and there lies ahead at least five and for many eight further years of training. Furthermore, these post-grad exams are not easy to navigate with a pass rate of often less than 50% of those who sit them.

It is usual to undertake exams with the Royal College that you wish to train in, but the College of Emergency Medicine didn't exist when I was going through the process, being founded only in 2008. At that time, if you wished to earn a place on an Emergency Medicine higher specialist training programme you had to pass either the Royal College of Physicians (RCP) or the Royal College of Surgeons (RCS) membership examinations. Having weighed up the options I embarked on the surgical route.

It was tough working in the ED on a rota in which you worked six out of eight weekends. Fifty-six hours a week didn't leave a lot of time for studying, not to mention getting married, but eventually after months of study and sacrificing evenings off, I flew to Newcastle upon Tyne to sit the exam. I struggled through both papers. Reading the first question, 'Which of the following structures go through the internal obturator foramen?' I knew there was no way I was going to pass this exam. This was detailed surgical anatomy of the hip not routinely encountered on an ED round. And so, it proved. When I opened the letter a few weeks later I had failed both. Experiences like this help you maintain perspective and keep you grounded.

Six months later, I found myself back once again pen in hand, this time at the Royal College of Surgeons in Ireland sitting four separate one-hour multiple choice papers: one anatomy, one physiology, one pathology and one practical surgical paper. I read the first question, 'Light adaptation takes longer than dark adaptation – true or false.' This was a far more positive start. I closed my eyes then opened them again and ticked false. Putting down my pencil at the end of the last exam I felt quietly confident. I hoped to have passed two. When I opened the letter a few weeks later and saw four passes, I felt an enormous sense of relief: I was ecstatic that I had regained some free time in the evenings and felt proud that I managed to pass Part 1 RCS membership without working in surgery. Over the next few years, further sets of exams followed, enabling me to advance to the final stage of specialist training as a registrar.

I interviewed for the Northern Ireland Accident and Emergency (A&E) higher specialist training programme twice and was unsuccessful both times. It was highly competitive. There were only two posts in the whole of the country and a lot of high-calibre candidates. The first time I was fourth. 'You did very well, but you are still young Jonny,' Mr Fee, who was on the panel, had reassured me afterwards, 'You just need more experience.' The second time I was more nervous – the stakes felt higher, but this interview did not go well. I knew I hadn't performed as I wanted or was capable and wasn't surprised therefore when I narrowly missed out again. But all the studying, all the shifts finishing at two o'clock in the morning, all those weeks of working nights were beginning to feel futile. It appeared doors were closing in front of me once more and I didn't know what my next move should be. Chatting things through with Heather I decided to look further afield and applied to various jobs in London, Leeds, Manchester and Bristol that offered a five-year Emergency Medicine higher specialist training rotation, but I didn't really want commit to relocating for that length of time. It was then I spotted a job advert for a one-year post at the University Hospitals of Leicester A&E Department. This was perfect. I would be working at a higher level, but it would only be for one year and would afford me one further opportunity to interview for the Northern Ireland scheme. My older brother Peter lived about an hour away so there was the bonus of being able to spend more time with him and his family.

A month or so later I opened a letter informing me that I had been shortlisted. On the journey to the interview I sat back looking out the window. I knew very little about Leicester and the only associations that sprung to mind were Gary Lineker, the former England footballer, and Walker's Crisps! As we entered deeper into the city, I saw a sign for the King Power Stadium where Leicester City Football Club play, and shortly afterwards we passed the Leicester Tigers Rugby Club. It relaxed me a little. Surely, I could make a home in a city with such a rich history of sport. As it transpired this was to be tested when the next day I took a phone call informing me I had been successful.

Four months later Heather and I moved to a small village about four miles south of Leicester. It was hard leaving family and friends, to move to where we knew no one.

The University Hospitals of Leicester A&E department was the busiest in the UK, the third busiest in Europe and the fifth busiest in the world. The pathology that I got to see every day was staggering and it was a great experience.

Later that year, I interviewed one final time for the Northern Ireland training scheme. When I was unsuccessful for the third time, I couldn't bring myself to ask where I had been placed. This time I accepted that the door had well and truly been closed and made peace to change our long-term plans and set aside my preformed expectations.

Around this time A&E Departments were renamed as Emergency Departments in the hope that it would deter people attending with minor complaints and reduce the workload for the staff. Departments were getting busier year on year and days of having time to sit down and rest during a night shift were over, but though the work in Leicester was high in intensity I had settled well. The whole ED team had been immediately welcoming and Leicester was increasingly feeling like home. Four months later I interviewed and was appointed to the East Midlands Emergency Medicine Higher Specialist Training Programme. After all the anguish I was finally, officially starting my training as a registrar to become an Emergency Medicine consultant: this new title and new start felt good.

The next four years passed in a haze. A busy shift pattern, more exams and a new baby didn't leave much time for anything else and in 2008 after what felt like a marathon, I completed my exams to become a Fellow of College of Emergency Medicine, enabling me to finally apply for jobs as an ED consultant. I was delighted to be appointed in Leicester and after many years of investment was looking forward to beginning to finally find some stability.

In 2012, I expanded this role taking on the post of medical education lead in the ED. This meant that in addition to undergraduate education of medical students I was involved in developing and implementing teaching programmes for all levels of ED trainees in our department. A year earlier I had commenced a master's in medical education through the University of Dundee. This was a distance degree, undertaken online. I did not have to commute to Scotland, but it was another significant commitment of time. By now I was thirty-seven years old and had been studying for much of the twelve years following graduation, in addition to working brutal ED shift systems. We had two young children and life was busy. When I was on call I worked from six o'clock in the evening to one o'clock in the morning. I then had to decide whether the department was under control and safe for me to go home for the registrars to manage until eight o'clock the next morning. Sometimes it could be three or four in the morning before things were stable and I was confident to leave. Even when I did, most of the time I left with the full understanding that I could be called back in at any point in the middle of the night. I distinctly recall a night I had returned home and was just unlocking the front door when I was alerted. Four people were coming in who had been stabbed. The door hadn't even got opened and I was still in the department by eight o'clock the next morning when the day team arrived, and I was expected to be starting another day's work. On call was especially tiring when you had a young family who didn't account for the hour that you finally slipped into bed.

The prospect in these circumstances of embarking on yet more studying required careful consideration and support. There reaches the point where you just want to come home from work and relax, watch TV, eat a takeaway and enjoy time with your family. But because I enjoyed the educational role so much and was keen to develop it further, Heather and I both felt it was a necessary commitment to expand my learning and improve my qualifications.

Thursday was my day off from the ED, so I sat every week and worked through all the modules in each section. The process of achieving my master's involved first completing a postgraduate certificate in medical education, then a diploma and finally my master's dissertation.

There was a medical education concept when I was training which was: see one, do one, teach one. Over the years this fell out of favour as it evidently takes more than one attempt to become competent in a skill and there are many of them to learn. It was replaced by practising skills in a simulated environment. It is now possible to suture on a square piece of artificial skin, insert a cannula into a moulded plastic arm or even insert a catheter into an artificial penis until you feel confident and competent to do it for real. Simulation also became the standard way to train for the management of cardiac arrest and trauma in both adults and children with specific courses that had been designed to achieve this. Aligned with my role in ED, I was trained as an instructor on these national courses so was familiar with the development and increasing use of simulation.

Practicality, safety and flexibility meant extension into the sphere of assessment became inevitable and today almost all medical examinations at both undergraduate and postgraduate level utilise simulation. Previously these had entailed assessing real patients, but this was logistically difficult, tiring for those already unwell and difficult to standardise. Objective structured clinical examinations or OSCEs are now the most common method employed assessing clinical skills in a timed period with a predetermined, scripted scenario.

During my work as undergraduate lead in the department I developed a particular interest in constructing these and over time was given the responsibility to introduce, plan and implement an OSCE circuit at the end of each training block in the ED. This consisted of twelve stations that lasted ten minutes each, where a student was assessed on focused clinical skills such as history taking, physical examination, diagnosis, communication and counselling. I really enjoyed this aspect of my job and over time began to write more complicated ED stations to be used in the Finals OSCE. The beauty was this role provided scope for imagination and afforded an opportunity for creativity. Two years later I was appointed lead for the Finals OSCE at University of Leicester Medical School with responsibility to oversee the whole end of course practical exam, covering all specialities not just ED. There were many aspects to the role. The exam had to be designed to be fair and balanced, the OSCE stations needed to be written and then practised: firstly to ensure that they achieved the goals intended and secondly that there was sufficient time in the station to accomplish them. Finally, the whole process had to be standardised and part of this was ensuring the examiners understood their roles.

In this capacity I arranged for a series of examiner blooper scenarios to be recorded in the purpose-built exam centre, which could be set up to mimic the bays on a ward with four areas separated by a curtain. There was a hospital bed with a whiteboard above them, a bedside cabinet, a chair and a table. We had emailed a request for help to volunteer examiners, simulated patients and final-year medical students. We recorded twelve in total, but I had a particular favourite. We recorded a mock student's first OSCE station. A bell rang after ten minutes to indicate that her time was up and that she had completed the station. 'That is the end of the station. You must stop now,' the mock examiner instructed, gesturing for the student to leave the bay and move on to the next one which was beside the one they had just completed. The curtains were flimsy, so the examiners had been instructed not to talk about the student's performance after they had left. In this video the student was outside the station but, through the closed curtain, could audibly hear the examiner lean over to the simulated patient and say, 'She wasn't very good,' and shaking his head, added, 'I don't know what the medical school is doing these days!' The student looked distraught and would have had eleven further stations to complete after this. This mock OSCE station demonstrated how a throw away comment that wasn't intended to be heard had a massive impact on the student, affecting her confidence for the rest of the OSCE. Words matter, and they should be chosen wisely or sometimes not at all.

When I was diagnosed my immediate determination was to keep all the various work plates spinning both in the ED and medical school. I considered that in the long term I would find the educational role easier to sustain with symptom progression, particularly as ED work involves so many practical procedures, so I decided to persevere with the original plan. Within a month of being diagnosed I was made an honorary associate professor in medical education and six months later I submitted my master's dissertation which considered how medical students who performed well in exams self-regulate. It had been a real struggle to complete it. My symptoms were not stabilised, and I was still struggling with significant fatigue. On many occasions it was hard to focus, meaning everything took longer than it had before. But I had come so far and didn't want three years of invested work to be wasted so I persevered until it was completed. However, it was a significant sacrifice of family time, and I couldn't have done it without Heather's support. When I graduated with a distinction it assured me that I was still able to work at a high standard even if it had been challenging and reinforced my decision to continue working.

Around this time the General Medical Council (GMC) had begun to implement standardisation across all medical schools, establishing national criteria for the professional exams which directly contributed to the award of a medical degree. This was a new development in medical education and processes needed to be developed to not only train examiners so they would all mark to the same standard, but to also address situations that had arisen over the years due to examiner behaviour that disadvantaged students. In 2019 (and three years after diagnosis), I became an associate at the GMC, as one of the team leaders helping to oversee this work.

I once believed that perseverance was demonstrated when grit and determination resulted in the successful attainment of a long-term goal or objective. But the path of the past twenty years has persuaded me that it is more nuanced than I previously considered. Undoubtedly, the previous is an example of perseverance but is not the only way it manifests. Perseverance is less about reaching an endpoint as maintaining forward momentum towards one. Sometimes this involves changing the destination when the way to an original destination is blocked, on every path attempted. I had pursued several options that would lead to a career in general practice but found my way repeatedly thwarted. To keep moving forwards required willingness to alter predetermined plans and openness to consider other possibilities. Other times it required discovery of a different path leading to the same destination. Nowhere had a relocation to England featured in my original plans but when the most obvious track in Northern Ireland had been frustrated, I had to broaden my horizons and extend the limit of possibilities to maintain the plan of completing specialist training in Emergency Medicine. But finally, there are occasions when what we need is to get a shovel and work hard to clear the landslide that has blocked our way. There was only one way to pass my exams and complete my master's – increase the hours of study, complete more questions, learn more facts. Discipline and hard work were requisite.

All of these reflect perseverance, but deciding which is the best option in a particular situation isn't always easy. This highlights the link between perseverance and learning. There are occasions when it seems as though the path is leading us backwards and it can feel both demoralising and disappointing. But we are still further forward for what we have learnt. I love mazes but it is rarely possible to get to the centre on the first attempt. It usually involves walking a path to discover a blind end, before turning and retracing our steps. But the next time we know to take a different option. Every dead end informs us and leads us closer to the right path, and part of the eventual joy in reaching the end is because of the challenge in getting there.

Adapting to change is rarely a linear process but a cycle characterised by successes and failures in which we sometimes move backward as well as forward. The biggest enemy to adaptability is not moving in a wrong direction it is becoming stuck so we don't move at all.

The first step in overcoming inertia is difficult. When, despite my best intentions, I have found myself stuck it is perseverance, aided by helping hands that helped generate the power to haul my feet from out of the sinking sand. But isn't easy. Perseverance, like a muscle, is developed and strengthened when it is loaded and placed under strain, and arguably one of the biggest loads is dealing with loss.

CHAPTER 7

The ED with PD

Increasing my levels of physical activity represented an effort to keep at bay the changes being imposed on my body by Parkinson's disease. I hated the feeling of stiffness and heaviness, and I wanted to do everything possible to lessen and slow their progress by pushing hard in the opposite direction. I knew the fitter I became, the more I raised the bar for my strength and flexibility, the further PD would have to advance to catch me. Sometimes the process of adapting to live better involves putting in place defences. Strengthening the ramparts, establishing surveillance and firing artillery all limit the progress of an opponent. And so it is with PD. Maximising health and fitness, careful monitoring for example of bowel habits and sleep to enable early intervention and proactive measures such as Vitamin D and calcium supplementation for bone health are all forms of defence. But sometimes resistance can be unhelpful and there are circumstances when what is needed to facilitate adaptation is the very opposite.

————————————

After the shock of my diagnosis subsided, my thoughts very quickly turned to the implications for work. This was a big concern and occupied much of my thinking in the first few months. I was only 41 years old with a young family. How would Parkinson's affect us financially? Would we have to move house? How would I be able to help the kids if they went to university? Again, there were so many questions and no matter how many hours Heather and I spent chatting, many of them remained questions without answers.

I loved my job and the prospect of having to stop hung over my head like an ominous thundercloud. QUB has as its motto *'Pro tanto quid retribuamus'* which means *'For so much, what shall we give back?'* I have never forgotten the words. They motivated me 25 years ago and they continue to do so today. I have always considered it a privilege to serve my community in caring for and looking after the sick. So, the decision to return to work was a very easy one to make. Whether I would be able to continue working as I had before was less straightforward and complicated in part by the field of medicine in which I specialised.

By the time you become an ED consultant you are the most senior decision maker in the department. When you are on call or overseeing the 'shop floor' you are responsible for supervising all clinical decisions. The origins of an ED 'shop floor' stem from a traditional department store. It is a bustling environment, full of industry

DOI: 10.1201/9781003600671-7

with staff working hard to meet the many and varied needs of all those who have come through the door.

Resuscitation is one dimension of work in the ED, where those who are clinically deteriorating, unstable or critical are admitted. Majors is the area where patients present with an array of symptoms which can range from abdominal pain and headaches to psychiatric symptoms, pregnancy-related symptoms or post-operative complications. Not everyone will need to be admitted to hospital, but some will deteriorate and become critical if they are not seen quickly. Work in this area is about risk stratification, about identifying those low-risk cases that can go home and the high-risk cases who require timely intervention. Critical in managing this area is the ability to assess the big picture as well as the detail. This was a lesson I learnt right at the beginning of training. During one shift in majors, I had picked up the chart of the patient who was next to be seen. The presenting complaint was a little finger injury in a twenty-year-old male. These patients would normally be seen in minors but the triage nurse thought that he looked pale and his heart rate, at just over one hundred beats a minute, was faster than it should have been. When I walked into the cubicle I could tell immediately that something wasn't right: he looked as white as the sheet he was sitting on. I took the history and it transpired that he had fallen during a run and landed on some bricks. The laceration on his left little finger would need stitches. On examination, he had a few grazes on the left side of his abdomen and complained of some minor pain. I was worried that he may have injured his spleen when he fell and asked the nurses to check a urine sample for blood as a marker of possible abdominal injury. When it came back positive, I phoned the surgical registrar who reviewed and admitted him for observation. The next day he had an operation to remove a ruptured spleen. What a patient presents with may not be their only problem.

Minors is the area that largely deals with accidents. Patients attend with lacerations, sprains or broken bones. From fingers to toes, wrists to knees, ankles to hips, any joint could be affected – it is always busy but particularly so on a Saturday and Sunday afternoon. Finally, there is the Emergency Decisions Unit (EDU). In our department there are twelve beds and four ward-type chairs where patients are admitted on pathways pending further clinical assessment before deciding whether to admit or discharge them. This includes patients presenting with head injuries, alcohol dependence, mental health and back pain.

At any given point there are multiple staff working across the four sections of the department including nurses, doctors in training and increasingly advanced clinical practitioners (qualified nurses who have undergone a master's level degree course to enable them to assess and manage patients independently). Doctors in training change jobs every four or six months so there is a high turnover of staff, each one arriving at the bottom of a steep learning curve. The consultant needs to be available to answer and address any clinical queries or concerns any of those working may have and to oversee their decision making.

Supervision is a particularly stressful aspect of the job. It is impossible to review every patient yourself to make your own assessment. You need therefore to be constantly exercising judgement about the reliability of the information being presented to you whilst also trying to keep oversight of decisions by those not seeking help. It requires understanding of the variable competencies of the staff working – a task made harder by shift work. You may have encountered a particular member of staff only a few times before or never! When you make your round of the different areas of the ED to check on the staff, you are giving advice on not one or two cases but multiple cases: all involving assessing risk, each one of equal importance to that individual patient. Frequently I would turn from giving advice to discover a queue of four or five people waiting. Argos is the 'all-seeing' 100-eyed giant, from Greek mythology – any ED consultant would yearn for such vision.

The role of supervision also involves having your own train of thought and concentration constantly interrupted. One evening I was working in majors and was reviewing a patient with abdominal pain when I heard a shout for help from a nurse in the next bay. Her patient, who had been brought in with crushing central chest pain, had just arrested. Quickly apologising I left my own patient to join her. I confirmed cardiac arrest by feeling for a pulse and checking for breathing, but neither was present. We started CPR, one of the nurses commenced chest compressions and I ventilated via a bag-valve-mask attached to fifteen litres of oxygen. We attached him to the defibrillator pausing to check his rhythm. He was in ventricular fibrillation, which is unsustainable with life, but which can respond to an electrical shock. Switching to automatic pilot we worked according to protocol and delivered one.

After two minutes of CPR we observed that the patient had started to breathe on his own and had a weak but palpable pulse. I shouted at him, 'Can you hear me John, can you hear me?' He started to blink and slowly opened his eyes. It must be a strange feeling opening your eyes after your heart has stopped with a group of faces peering down on you. We were relieved when he opened his mouth and asked, 'Are you from Belfast?' and smiled at each other knowing he was neurologically intact, having recognised my accent. Quick intervention had prevented his brain being starved of oxygen, however there was no time to enjoy the moment. As soon as the management plan had been given for transfer to coronary care it was straight back to the patient I had abandoned, to pick up where I had left off. There is nothing extraordinary in this; it's the day-to-day reality of what we do.

In addition to supervision, you are also responsible for helping to manage the flow of patients through the department, to limit waiting times and create beds for those still in ambulances. There is a constant monitoring of screens to see how many patients have arrived each hour and how long they are waiting to be seen, and the process doesn't end with assessment. We also need to know who has already been assessed and is waiting to go to the wards to ensure that everything has been done to facilitate their progress and make certain they are receiving ongoing treatment until they are admitted.

To work in ED is to live life on the edge and requires a calm mind and steady hands. It involves multitasking on a minute-by-minute basis and working in the knowledge that every wrong decision has potential to cause harm or even death. No shift is predictable, and there are so many uncontrollable variables and colossal emotional strain. We are witnessing horrific injuries and dealing with unexpected deaths across all ages and can finish a shift feeling deeply traumatised to have to get up and do it all again the next day. We are managing stressful situations with limited resources and whilst this is all outweighed when a life is saved or when you tell a spouse, partner, mother or father that their loved one is going to be ok, it remains an intense and pressured environment in which decision making is unrelenting from the start of an eight-hour shift until the end. The ability to constantly and rapidly shift focus of attention is essential, as is cognitive flexibility, which necessitates precision and attention to detail on the one hand, and strategic oversight of the big picture on the other.

By 2016, I had been working as an Emergency Medicine consultant for seven years, spending four days a week in the ED and one day a week at the medical school, and although it was hard work, I loved it. So, when I was informed of my diagnosis at clinic and signed off work for four weeks, it was my immediate intention to return as soon as possible. Being an ED doctor was an important part of my identity and I was not ready to give it up. Obviously, I understood that the time would come when I would not be able to continue work but I didn't consider that point had been arrived at. My symptoms were mild and although I was aware of them, they were at this stage less obvious to my colleagues and patients. But I had to accept that there was a cost. Whilst I was still able to filter and process complex information, sustain concentration and multitask, it required more effort and used much more energy than it had before. Each shift was leaving me exhausted, and I had become increasingly aware I was running close to empty.

The time signed off acted as an important break. It provided opportunity for rest, perspective and space, all of which were necessary in determining the right path forward. Left to my own devices I would have probably ploughed on and returned to work much sooner, but I am glad of the wisdom of my consultant and family to insist on it. It taught me an important lesson that you can't be your own physician. It isn't always possible to see the wood from the trees when you are exhausted and emotionally invested. You may know all the right information but weighing it up correctly is another matter, and in the beginning I didn't understand what the implications of the disease would be for my work because I didn't really understand Parkinson's as a condition.

On the one hand I wanted to avoid risk and be ahead of the ball in ensuring that when I eventually stopped work I would do so still functioning at the highest standard. But, on the other hand I knew I was still capable of contributing and was worried about making decisions based on fear and the possibility of what might happen in the future, rather than the evidence of the present. I recognised that decisions once taken would be very difficult to undo, and I did not want to regret having acted too soon.

In such circumstances there is great value in objectivity and at this stage I desperately needed it. Occupational Health were instrumental in helping me become unstuck. Apart from the occasional missed shift due to the flu or odd migraine, I had never been off work for a significant period, so even the simple practicality of navigating sick notes and hospital referrals was a steep learning curve, but they guided and supported me through the decision-making process and I am very grateful for their input. They liaised with my neurologist and suggested, in the first instance, some adjustments to the nature and pattern of work which would enable me to keep functioning at a high level and continue to add value to the team. I would continue all the clinical responsibilities of an ED consultant as before. However, they suggested that my clinical work should be focused primarily in the mornings in a fixed pattern and with no on call, and though I would still work one in every eight weekends, it would again only be in the mornings. My departmental administration work of investigating incidents and giving a medico-legal opinion to the trust would be reduced, and attendance at both the large weekly departmental meeting and the consultant meeting would become flexible and at the discretion of my symptoms.

Removing my on call with no work after six o'clock in the evening made a massive difference. Stress is a huge dopamine burner, and a large amount of mine dissipated overnight by making that simple adjustment. For the first time since graduation, life developed predictable routines. With time, I would come to see just how important routine is when you are living with Parkinson's. All these significantly helped my fatigue and I noticed an improvement in non-motor symptoms, enabling me to return everyday.

However, it became clear over the following year that two areas of the ED were exacerbating my Parkinson's symptoms. Despite having my medication tweaked I needed to take three months off in 2018 as I was struggling to work effectively in the main ED and was finding that I didn't have anything left in the tank when I got home.

The first was working in resus. I noticed that managing the sickest patients, running a trauma team, managing an aggressive or violent patient and undertaking procedural sedation were increasing my symptoms, leaving me feeling stiff down my whole left side.

Decision making in this area, as outlined, is not only time critical and high stakes but relentless. On one shift a trauma patient with a fracture-dislocation of their right ankle had arrived and they needed to have it pulled back into place and plastered under what was called procedural sedation. With the help of one of the ED registrars we started oxygen, inserted an intravenous cannula and gained consent for what we needed to do. As we titrated the painkillers and the sedation medications through the cannula the patient gradually became drowsy. It is a balance to find the sweet spot where they are neither under-sedated nor over-sedated, as in the latter their airway would be at risk as it wasn't protected. The ED nurses had prepared the plaster that would need to be applied after we had relocated the ankle but it would require moulding. The ED registrar got into position to provide counter traction, and I got into position at the foot of the bed, supporting the ankle and leg in my hands. I nodded and called to pull. One, two, three . . . we gave it a huge pull but it was very stiff and did not immediately relocate. We pulled again and this time it popped straight back into place, but the patient let out the loudest shriek! As I stood holding the relocated right ankle waiting for the nurses to apply the plaster, I could see my left hand and foot visibly tremoring. I don't think anyone noticed but I felt awful; the stress had used up a lot of dopamine and left me symptomatic. When we finished, I had just washed my hands when the red phone rang, and I was informed a trauma patient was arriving in five minutes.

Stress is the enemy of PD. From the dim and distant past of biochemistry lectures at medical school I recalled that adrenaline is derived from noradrenaline, which in turn is derived from dopamine. In the ED we thrive on adrenaline. We run on adrenaline. It is impossible to work in an environment like resus without it. However, this inevitably depletes dopamine levels, so much so that in certain situations the environment was directly responsible for the emergence of symptoms which were otherwise not present at any other time. Furthermore, dopamine was not only depleted in the areas of the brain needed for movement but also in areas of my brain regulating emotion and executive function, leading me to feel anxious, unfocused and distracted and at times unmotivated and apathetic, not how anyone wants to be feeling in the middle of a busy shift. ED doctors may thrive on adrenaline, but it turns out that ED doctors with PD do not.

The second environment that was becoming problematic was the Children's Emergency Department. During my higher specialist training I had undertaken an additional year of training in Paediatric Emergency Medicine, and as a consultant, twenty-five percent of my clinical work was in this area. However, I noticed I was becoming particularly symptomatic when I was treating a crying or screaming child, especially if I had to insert a cannula into their veins and take some blood samples. I became aware of parents noticing when my left hand started to tremor during procedures.

It was at this point I had to make a hard decision. I could have continued pushing myself to the limit, but I knew it was simply delaying the inevitable and I did not want to jeopardise my ability to sustain work in the long term by failing to act when I noticed the creeping impact of PD on my work. I don't think anyone knows with complete certainty the 'right' time for decisions like these. They are profoundly personal and therefore difficult to generalise. Self-awareness and intuition play important roles. But, as far as I could be certain, I felt that I had reached an important turning point, so I made an appointment with both Occupational Health and my line managers to discuss further adjustments. This time the outcomes were far more consequential in the decision to stop working in the most acute and critical situations of resus, majors and the paediatric department.

I would be lying if I didn't admit this was a huge body blow, and eight years later I still feel it as a loss. These were areas that I loved working in the most, and having to give them up was a bitter pill to swallow. I felt angry that after all the many years of training, the capacity to treat the sickest patients was being taken away from me just as I felt I was reaching my prime. My whole identity was shaken to the core. How could I call myself an Emergency Medicine doctor when I didn't see emergencies? But I was very fortunate that our department has an EDU. It provided many advantages in helping me to manage my Parkinson's. The patients in EDU had already been seen, risk assessed and started on treatment if needed. I could take planned breaks, and it is a slower pace than the main department. With support from colleagues and agreement of the trust I have been able to shift to additional departmental administration and continue clinical work in a less critical environment. However, I miss being there and will occasionally walk through resus, majors and children's just to remind myself.

In managing a progressive condition there are times when change can be resisted and we can take measures to push back against it and limit its progress. However, there are other occasions when despite intervention and the best of efforts it results in loss. Ask those who live with PD and they will describe a myriad of things they can no longer do. I can't spend a morning shopping in town without having to abandon Heather several times to find a toilet; I can no longer eat only when I want or when I'm hungry but according to my medication schedule, or have a lie in past 6 am – even on summer holidays. Some losses are small and adjusted to relatively easily, but others take much longer to process. Furthermore, they often encompass more than just function, impacting identity, confidence, self-worth and social connections.

Whilst the first instinct might be to fight or deny such change it eventually becomes imperative to accept it, to enable the process of adaptation to proceed. But yet again there is no set formula, and this will look different from individual to individual. Some find the hardest aspect is to move beyond denial, others get stuck in anger and for some apathy becomes the main roadblock. It is also important to bear in mind that there is no single process of grief. Rather in progressive conditions there is a perpetual process of adjusting to multiple losses over a long period, and at any given moment I have been in several different stages of loss at the same time. Some losses are grieved and quickly processed, others take years and even then they leave a permanent imprint. Giving up aspects of my work was certainly felt as a loss. However, I recognised, with help, that sometimes I was going to need to concede a battle to win the war. I did not want to stop but at the same time understood that finishing in these pressured environments would enable me to live well by sustaining work for a much longer period. This was adaptation by concession. It was gaining by letting go.

CHAPTER 8

More Medication

Levodopa has been used in the management of PD since the 1960s. Although I yearn for the development of disease-modifying drugs (DMD) that will alter the course of this condition, I am mindful that sometimes my frustration at not having what I long for can make me lose sight of what I already have. Before its introduction as the gold standard, patients with Parkinson's in hospital were often so stiff that they had to be transported on flat boards. Today, I am very grateful that all the medications I am prescribed exist and for the role levodopa plays in maintaining my function. Looking back less than a century, life for someone with Parkinson's was very different, and if afforded the opportunity I would not choose to time travel back to then. However, in the beginning my feelings towards levodopa were more ambivalent.

Just as an off-chance attempt at Bollywood dancing led to my diagnosis, it was a simple encounter that initiated the discussion about starting it. I was walking up the hospital corridor with an ED colleague, on the way to a meeting, when she enquired, 'What happened to your leg? Have you injured it?' I was a little taken aback. I hadn't even been aware that I was walking abnormally and yet the signs of my Parkinson's were sufficiently evident to have induced concern in her.

Not long before this happened Heather and I had decided to change consultant care. We did so because I was struggling to be a patient. I suspect this is a common experience amongst healthcare professionals who find themselves on the other side of the consultation desk. We are trained to review test results, reach decisions and recommend treatments, and it was not easy for me to shift to the opposite dynamic in the patient–doctor relationship; to receive advice rather than give it. When the consequences are personal, we want to see our scans and study the evidence, and it is hard to relinquish control. I was instinctively trying to be my own doctor. But of course, as soon as we become the patient, we lose our sense of clinical objectivity and we need others to provide it. My struggle was perpetuated by the fact I had decided to continue working in both the ED and medical school and was therefore frequently interacting with my consultant on a professional level. I felt embarrassed and self-conscious especially as I began to realise there was far more about PD that I didn't understand than I did. The decision to move out of area, to a new consultant who I did not know and who had expertise in movement disorders, represented an important turning point. For the first time since I had been diagnosed, I felt able to remove the mantle that accompanies those two small letters 'Dr' in front of my name and to walk into the clinic as 'Jonny.' Conscious of a weight lifted, it was liberating to discover that

DOI: 10.1201/9781003600671-8

I not only needed but wanted to be guided in treatment, and as I metaphorically took off my white coat and set down my stethoscope, I tried for the first time not to be a patient doctor or a doctor patient, but just a patient.

The first appointment with my new consultant happened to take place a week or so after my colleague had commented on my walking. This was the first time I was conscious that those who did not know me could identify a problem, and it bothered me, so having an opportunity to discuss my concerns was helpful. During this consultation my new consultant pulled up the images from my dopamine transporter (DAT) scan on his monitor and started to explain in a simple, straightforward way what it showed. He told me that the loss of the dopaminergic receptors was greater on the right than on the left. (The brain is wired in such a way that neurons cross over and the right side of the brain is responsible for movement on the left and vice versa, so that made perfect sense to me as my symptoms were worse on my left.) He went on to explain that although I was presently symptomatic on my left side, there was sufficient change on the scan to indicate progression to the right would follow in due course. How quickly that would happen, like so many aspects of this condition, was uncertain. I told him about the incident in the corridor and discussed my fears and concerns.

'Why do I feel so lousy and exhausted?' I asked. 'Because you are very undermedicated,' he immediately replied. 'Having looked at your scan, you are going to need a hefty dose of medication to get you moving again.' He explained the rationale and thinking behind his philosophy to maximise and maintain function by treating symptoms aggressively. He felt that rasagiline was providing inadequate control and that it was the right time to introduce levodopa. Before I left clinic he prescribed anti-sickness medication for three days, along with oral levodopa (Sinemet).

I found the decision to commence levodopa surprisingly difficult to process. I am not entirely sure why, but I think it was because it signified a point of no return. I knew once it was started that it wouldn't be stopped. This was for life. When I was first commenced on rasagiline I had also hoped it would buy me time and maybe delay the start of levodopa for a few years, but it did not bring any meaningful improvement. The decision to begin levodopa therefore represented my first experience of treatment failure and felt like concrete evidence that my disease was not as mild as I had hoped. I was no longer playing in the shallow waters of PD; I had to face the diagnosis full on. However, my initial reluctance soon passed as the medication took effect. After one week I felt as though I had been recharged like a battery, noting a particular improvement in my levels of fatigue. But it required several further reviews to improve management of my motor symptoms.

It is very difficult when you live with a chronic progressive condition to monitor and measure improvement in symptoms. I imagine many think that being a doctor makes the task easier, but I have not found this so. Change happens in small increments and is difficult to quantify. Assessment of Parkinson's symptoms is subjective, and I have discovered that even my own personal judgement varies depending on the relative balance of non-motor symptoms at the time. If I am feeling particularly fatigued or have high levels of anxiety my perception of motor symptoms is always much worse. Moreover, there is a natural degree of fluctuation in symptoms throughout the course of a day and from one day to the next. Often, I find myself questioning whether I am feeling worse because there has been some permanent progression or because of factors which are reversible. Have I simply been pushing it too hard in the gym or am I overtired because of an especially stressful period at work? When such questions begin to occupy your thinking, it becomes very easy to develop hyper-vigilance. I was starting to monitor every minor variation, seeking to determine the reason for it. This pattern of overthinking quickly destroyed all enjoyment of the present and left me feeling mentally wiped out. Furthermore, it was futile, as no amount of thinking or analysis could provide concrete answers. In short, the process of determining whether there has been a change can be difficult and feels stressful, and when I attend review appointments I do not look forward to having to answer the question 'How have you been?' because the honest answer is, 'I don't really know.' Some days are good, others not, and in truth it's hard to keep track.

A few years ago I was invited to participate in a trial for a smartwatch known as a Personal KinetiGraph or PKG. Whilst such technology has limitations, I do feel there is benefit in attempting to objectively track symptoms. Tracking doesn't change symptoms, but it can alter our ability to manage conditions. Recording data can, over time, help to normalise symptoms if they are part of everyday experience. Furthermore, when you know symptoms are being tracked it relieves the pressure of trying to make sense of them in the immediate time frame. It is possible to become 'forgetful' from one day to the next, and to relax because evidence has been captured that will enable any trends or patterns to emerge. Some may argue it may lead to preoccupation with symptoms, but I discovered the opposite, that my symptoms receded to the background of my field of awareness rather than dominating the picture because I knew data was being recorded. This in turn allowed me to experience symptoms without being fixated on them because I wasn't having to understand them in that instant, freeing mental energy for other tasks and helping me to better enjoy the present moment.

We don't all think or process information the same way, and the longer we have been managing PD the more Heather and I have increasingly recognised the role our personality plays in the process of adaption and how what is sometimes a strength can in other circumstances be a weakness. I prefer to base decisions on the evidence of facts and objective measures rather than feeling or gut instinct, but that is hard when what you are managing are symptoms which are neither easily objectified nor quantified. Perhaps it was helpful that I did not have access to the information which was being tracked by the watch, otherwise I would have become preoccupied not with the symptoms but with the data! I also prefer to focus on what is in front of me in each minute dealing with situations as they arise without a lot of deliberation. If there is a job that needs doing, I would rather do it at once and not leave it until a 'better time.'

Heather on the other hand is adept at reflection, at maintaining oversight of the big picture and identifying patterns, especially those which are presenting slowly over a long time frame of months. So, after the trial ended and I had seen the benefit of not analysing every minor variation, we adapted how we approach clinic reviews and the inevitable question, 'How have you been doing?' I realised that if I talk to Heather about my concerns and symptoms as they occur, she instinctively and mentally tracks them into the big picture to identify if there are new trends that need addressed. These months taught me an important lesson in the process of adaptation – dependence on others. We can't be all things to ourselves. None of us possess all the skills or attributes necessary to function without assistance. I needed the objectivity of my consultant and the big picture oversight of Heather. Wisdom is to know when, how and from whom to seek the help we need. It is to understand that there is a balance between passivity and foolhardiness. The former offloads all responsibility to others, the latter none. Both will hinder the process of adaptation.

Within three months my neurologist had changed the levodopa (Sinemet) to another medication (Stanek), one which contained levodopa and an additional drug (entacapone) shown to improve movement. The main side effect of this tablet is to turn your urine orange. This is due to the bright red–coloured coating. The first time I witnessed the colour in the toilet bowl it looked like I had consumed a keg of an orange-coloured fizzy drink from Scotland. Three months later he recommended adding an oral dopamine agonist (ropinirole), instructing me to increase the dose every two weeks over a period of twelve weeks. It took five increases in dose to finally get my left arm to swing again, almost two years after I was diagnosed.

Dopamine agonists work differently from levodopa as they stimulate the dopamine receptors in the brain to produce more natural dopamine. The problem is that they stimulate not only the thirty percent or so neurons left in your substantia nigra, but also the neurons in other parts of the brain including those unaffected by PD. This can lead to harmful side effects due to excessive levels of dopamine.

'These tablets can cause impulsive behaviour,' the neurologist informed us, 'but not always and usually at higher doses,' he added.

Impulse control disorders are characterised by repeated engagement in a behaviour despite adverse consequences. This is often proceeded by a feeling of increased internal tension, relieved by the behaviour, with diminished ability to resist it. People prescribed dopamine agonists have developed a range of compulsions including hypersexuality, gambling, overeating and shopping.

The consultant proceeded to advise Heather to monitor my internet use both in terms of content and time spent on my laptop. He suggested restricting and limiting snacks and recommended that she should have access to monitor all bank accounts, looking out for increased purchases or evidence of overspending. This was good advice, as the consequences of impulse control are potentially devastating. They can put strain on relationships, create dysfunction in the family and cause psychological harm, financial difficulty and ultimately isolation. Something I understood only too well.

'We will go to Dublin on one condition; I don't want you to drink,' I had said to Dad. It was a bright spring morning in 1993. As an eighteen-year-old, in my penultimate year at school, I thought I was doing the right thing. It must have pained him to hear as he knew what the implications were. 'Ok, I can do that,' he responded.

He had been drinking for years. I first suspected something was wrong when we started to go for a walk into town in the evening and he would disappear telling me that he just had to nip into the pub to speak to some of his friends. I stood outside as a twelve-year-old waiting, not daring to question it. Some nights he was away longer than others. When he returned, we walked back to the car and drove home.

Dad worked as a bank manager and had just been transferred to work in a town about eighty miles away. It meant the whole family needed to relocate. Peter, my older brother, and I had been given places at the local grammar school to start in September, but we had been unable to sell our house which would have allowed everyone to move together. The decision was reached that Dad, Peter and I would move and stay in a guest house a few miles away from our new school whilst Mum and my younger brother Tim remained until the house was sold. And so the family was split from a Sunday to Friday evening. On the drive back on Sunday night we always called into a local restaurant about halfway through our journey. I looked forward to stopping as I always got a coke. Dad drank what I thought was lemonade as it was clear. The odd thing was it didn't have any bubbles like mine. He always had a pickled egg from the jar after that. Even now if I close my eyes I can still remember how strong the smell of those were. For every pickled egg that was bought each week, I was bought a pack of Tayto Cheese and Onion crisps. It wasn't until the following summer that we were all able to move as a family.

Things continued to escalate particularly in the year before I departed to go to America. Maybe that's why I was so keen to apply, perhaps I just wanted breathing space and to escape. We would often find empty vodka bottles hidden at the bottom of the trees in the garden. I borrowed his golf bag one day and when I went to take out a new ball I found an empty bottle of triple distilled Smirnoff. It wasn't lemonade he was drinking after all. I would return home late from the cinema one Friday night to find him on the floor of the downstairs toilet unable to stand. I felt helpless. All I could do was to go and get a blanket and wrap it around him so he didn't get cold. Eventually a crisis point was reached. One night I returned late from a party and was climbing the stairs as quietly as possible so not to wake anyone. I had worked out a route that avoided all the stairs that creaked. I had just reached the top when I heard him call out to me to come to his room. As I opened the door he asked, 'Do you think my marriage is over?' A lump appeared in my throat: I knew that things were beyond repair, as mum had spoken to me only a few days before. I felt sorry for both of them as I replied, 'Yes, I think so but you'll need to ask Mum.' As a parent, you try and protect your children as much as you can, but when the family structure breaks down that protection is prone to developing cracks, and if it continues then gaping holes appear. After the family split Dad started to go to Alcoholics Anonymous (AA), which is an organisation that helps people who have become addicted to alcohol. After a few months of receiving help, his GP arranged for him to be admitted to a local hospital to undergo detox. I recall visiting him on the ward the day I had passed my driving test. He tried so hard to stop and so many times.

When I arrived at Dad's house that March morning in 1993, I was relieved to see that he was up and dressed and had opened the door. We had decided to take the train as it would be less tiring. I drove to the nearest station about twenty minutes away and we bought two return tickets. When we climbed on board, he needed a helping arm to get him onto the train. We had two seats at one of the tables in the coach and were surrounded by Irish rugby fans directly opposite us and four more at the table to the right of us. They were in great spirits and had every intention of enjoying themselves as they cracked open their six packs of beers. 'Would you like one?' they gestured to us both. As Dad shook his head, I said, 'No, thank you. We are alright.' The rest of the journey to Dublin was uneventful and we arrived at Connolly Station right on time. It was Six Nations Day and Dublin was bustling. Ireland had already lost to Scotland at Murrayfield and to France at home but had beaten Wales at Cardiff Arms Park, leaving them with two points out of a possible six. We were about to play England who had won two of their matches so far in the championship and were looking to make it three.

The atmosphere in Dublin on a match day is always one of anticipation and excitement and we decided to walk the short distance down to the DART, which is the city's overground metro system. Lansdowne Road was unique as the DART ran right under one of the stands. On one side of the railway track was the main stand and on the other side were the concrete pillars that supported it. As we walked down towards the stop I noticed Dad's hands were becoming shaky. 'Are you OK?' I asked. 'Yes, I just need to go in here for a minute or so.' I turned around and saw the sign 'Slattery's' one of Dublin's oldest pubs. As I watched him enter, I couldn't bear to follow him, so just as I had done six years previously, I stood outside and waited. 'You promised,' I said, when he reappeared. 'I know,' he replied, 'but I've only had one.' We agreed that there would be no more for the rest of the day.

We had to take a few rests as we walked down to the DART. His mobility wasn't as good as it used to be, and he appeared fearful. Of what I wasn't sure. As we waited for the train, I ate the packed lunch that I had made for both of us but he barely touched his. The match was thrilling to watch and I was on the edge of my seat throughout. There is always banter during the press build-up. England were supremely confident and were certain they were going to win. But that day they underestimated Ireland. Never underestimate an Irishman, and if you do make sure it's not fifteen of them. Ireland recorded a famous 17–3 win.

After the match as we made our way towards the DART station we were separated by the crowds. I could see Dad ahead but he couldn't see me. He started panicking and began frantically looking around to find me, shouting my name loudly in desperation. I pushed my way towards him and grabbed his arm locking it firmly with mine. 'I don't feel well,' he admitted.

We made it to the DART station, and with the money I had left in my wallet I hailed a taxi to Connolly Station. When we arrived, I helped Dad out and paid the fare. I didn't have a mobile phone back then and needed to make a phone call to one of my friends as I was due to go to an eighteenth birthday party later that evening. As I stood in the queue waiting for a public phone to become free, I heard a loud shriek behind me. Turning, I watched Dad collapse onto the floor. He was shaking all over, foaming at the mouth and turning blue. All I could do was shout for help. A member of staff radioed someone to call an ambulance and a very kind doctor who was in the station rushed over and opened his airway and told me that he was having a seizure. It seemed to continue for a lifetime, as did the wait for the ambulance, but in reality it lasted less than five minutes and ended just as the paramedics walked up the stairs. An oxygen mask was put on his face, a cannula was inserted into his arm, and he was placed on a stretcher and loaded into the back of an ambulance. With sirens blaring we raced across Dublin to the nearest Emergency Department. When we arrived, Dad was taken into resus and I had to wait outside. About forty-five minutes later the doctors came out to say that he had had a seizure secondary to alcohol withdrawal. They said it was dangerous for someone dependent on alcohol not to drink and asked when his last drink had been. 'About ten o'clock this morning,' I replied. They looked at their watches, it was now just after seven. 'That's probably why he's had the seizure then,' they said.

I felt horrendous, so guilty. I blamed myself for inducing the seizure by making it clear I was only going if he didn't drink. The doctors informed me he was being admitted as he was so confused. They thought it was best that I should try and return home. I went in to see him, kissed him on the forehead and walked out the door of the hospital. I had no idea where I was and no money, so I just started to run. I ran and ran and ran, through the streets of Dublin, occasionally stopping to ask passers-by for directions to Connolly Station. Slowly the landmarks became familiar. When I began to encounter Irish fans celebrating in the streets, I knew I wasn't far away.

Finally, I reached the station. On the train I sat and thought about all that had happened that day, how alcohol which started as a habit over the years had become an addiction. It had cost him his marriage, created dysfunction in the family and caused psychological harm to those closest to him, financial difficulty and ultimately isolation.

Six days later I was back in Dublin. Several months earlier I had put my name forward at school for the opportunity to be part of the crew of a tall ship. When my name was selected at random I couldn't wait to get on board. The *Asgard* was about to be my home for the next five days, a majestic ship with two main towering masts that we would be able to climb and release the sails when we were at sea. We had been paired with pupils from a school in Dublin and I was staying with Kieran and his family the night before we were to embark on our voyage. His parents were very welcoming. His dad was a cardiologist in the hospital where Dad had been brought to. I had phoned the hospital a few times during the week and knew that he was still an inpatient. Seeing him lying on the bed was distressing and upsetting, more so than when he had had the seizure. He looked at me with a puzzled look, as if he knew he should recognise me but his brain just couldn't process who I was. He eventually called me Paul, who was his younger brother. He didn't say anything that made any sense, and he was tremoring. I didn't stay long. Dad was never able to stop drinking altogether but after Dublin there were periods when he could reduce it or maintain abstinence, but ultimately, it always controlled him.

Despite his addiction, he was able to set up and build a successful local walking club. Fifty or sixty people would meet once a month, complete a predetermined walk and have a meal afterwards. He was an organiser and a people person at heart. He planned the routes and the menus and even dressed up as Santa for the Christmas Walk. He was extremely proud of all his sons, and he was able to control his drinking to attend my graduation and wedding. He was a good man, but alcohol took him down a road he couldn't get off.

I see a lot of alcohol dependence and alcohol withdrawal syndrome on my EDU ward rounds. I know now that it can occur within hours of stopping alcohol and it is treated by benzodiazepine administration based on symptoms that are present. Patients also need to be given intravenous vitamins as their levels are usually depleted. This protects against the progression of neuropsychiatric manifestations including confusion and hallucinations. I know now that Dad was dangerously unwell during that day in Dublin and in his subsequent time in hospital.

In the ED, I always spend as long as possible talking to every person with alcohol dependence before I refer them to our addictions team. I don't know if it helps but they know at least that someone has listened to them. You never know someone's backstory unless you ask. I recall speaking to a patient once who frequently attended our department. 'No one understands the pain,' he said. 'I never touched alcohol until I lost my wife twenty years ago.' He had swapped into a night shift to help a colleague and had a missed call from her at 03.22. He never could forgive himself when he returned home in the morning and found her dead. We always knew that Dad was not in a good way when the answering machine in his house was full and wouldn't let you leave a message. The morning the police found him dead on his bedroom floor I was torn by grief and relief that his nightmare had come to an end.

Back in clinic the neurologist continued his counsel. 'Make sure you have someone to confide in, someone who can inform us if there is a problem and we will reduce the dose,' he said. However, it struck me that by this point the horse may have already bolted and I was nervous to ensure my family history did not repeat itself.

Although my movement greatly improved with the combination of the new drug regime, it did indeed come at a cost. I was pleased that my arm swing had returned and was feeling great, but the increase in the dopamine agonist from 10 to 12 mg caused behavioural change. Within a few weeks my sex drive began to feel compulsive and over a few months it reached the point where what had always been intimate and enjoyable became associated with an unpleasant internal tension and feeling of pressure. It was causing strain to both of us, and at my next appointment the dopamine agonist was reduced. Within a few weeks, things had returned to normal, however there were other compulsive tendencies that continued to cause issues. I found I began snacking a lot. When the urge arose, despite them being hidden in the house I would drive down to my local supermarket or petrol station to buy some, at times eating them in the car even before I got home. Heather would often discover a stash of empty wrappers down the side of my car door, so in June 2018 my dopamine agonist tablet was changed to a twenty-four-hour patch, as the patch was associated with lower rates of impulsive control disorder (ICD).

There is a need to understand that managing chronic conditions is a dynamic process. There are many variables that influence outcomes, and these cannot always be controlled or predicted. Sometimes the only way to see what is round the corner is to look. If we insist on certainty of success beforehand then somewhere along the way we will become stuck. In this regard the concept of 'one step forward and two steps back' is an illusion, because you are always further forward for understanding and learning what doesn't work. So, although this period of impulse control problems was frustrating and unpleasant I do not regret trying and have peace of mind from not needing to wonder 'what if.' From a personal perspective it was also profoundly helpful in processing some of the emotions associated with Dad. When you love someone with addiction it is hard to avoid at least some degree of repressed anger, but my brief encounter with ICD provided some understanding of the hurdles Dad faced and the turmoil he suffered, helping to bring some healing.

CHAPTER 9

Connections and Coping

For the first two years I avoided seeking out others diagnosed with PD. The barrier was not a lack of opportunity. I had been signposted at clinic to a local support group run by Parkinson's UK but intentionally chose to avoid it, and the honest reason is that I was afraid of staring into the looking glass. It is one thing to read about symptoms in an information leaflet or textbook but another matter to observe them. I can learn that the tremor in PD is characteristically resting and pin-rolling or I can watch someone struggle with the basic task of drinking from a cup. Both teach me about tremor, but the former is academic and theoretical and the latter personal and visible.

It is hard to observe individuals with significant functional impairment without feeling something. It may be embarrassment, pity, compassion or admiration, but for anyone who has been told this is a projection of their own future there is almost certainly some element of fear. The truth is I didn't want to see those with more advanced disease in the early months after diagnosis because I found it emotionally overwhelming. I had to first work through the implications of the diagnosis in abstract before I could face them in 3D.

Being diagnosed with a progressive disease for which there is no cure or disease-modifying treatment explodes any illusion of infallibility. That sounds ridiculous because we all understand that we are not infallible. But if we are honest, many of us, especially in our younger decades, live as though we are. We make five- or ten-year plans until something like PD knocks us off balance in a powerful reminder that we are vulnerable: that nothing is certain and that there are things we cannot control. The instant I was diagnosed with PD all our carefully laid plans evaporated to be replaced by one huge question mark. Uncertainty became the new norm.

Initially this was both frightening and disorientating. It felt as though the ground beneath my feet had turned to sinking sand and, as months passed, I became increasingly stuck. I was desperate to move forward, I just wasn't sure how. With reflection my thinking was strongly influenced by the cohort of PD patients who are brought to the ED. Many are frail and dependent on others to help care for them and this had skewed my perception. There were many long conversations with Heather over coffee, and as we talked, I began to recognise that the biggest influence on my decision to avoid others were my own preconceptions of PD and disability in general.

At first, I didn't want to tell others because I was afraid that they would see me differently. But slowly I had to acknowledge that part of this was rooted in my own unconscious bias. It was not easy confronting the fact that the reason I was worried others would treat me differently was partly because I considered myself differently. After my diagnosis I viewed myself as 'less' than I had before. Less as a husband and father and less as a colleague. When I was thrust into the position of having to live with functional impairment rather than imagining what it was like, I started to understand that there were so many things I had misunderstood or not grasped at all. More than anything I had not considered the far-reaching impact it would have on my identity. To move forward I needed to stop feeling any sense of embarrassment or shame and find acceptance without diminishing the sense of who I was.

The first step was to deconstruct my own views of disability because they had proven to be on shaky foundations. I began to understand that by avoiding others with PD I was potentially robbing myself of the valuable insight they could provide and that any frameworks which I formed on my own would remain inadequate and insecure. What I needed at this stage was not best gleaned from a textbook or information leaflet but from the lived experience of others. I had to shift my focus from assimilating information to listening to others who had walked the same path, to learn from their mistakes and their successes, and to do this I needed to creep out from the shell of isolation in which I had taken refuge.

Once I had appreciated this, there were two groups of people with PD I was particularly keen to talk to. The first group were those with young onset Parkinson's disease (YOPD). This includes anyone diagnosed before the age of fifty. I suppose I was looking for people who were at a similar stage of life trying to maintain their work on the one hand, while raising a young family on the other. When I stopped avoiding and actively began to seek, I was surprised to discover it was easier to make connections than I had envisioned. Many of the charities have specific sections with information on YOPD, and there are an increasing number of groups both nationally and internationally that are specifically aimed at this cohort, such as Spotlight YOPD in the UK.

I found it hugely encouraging to read accounts of so many individuals living active, productive and enriched lives, working in jobs and their communities, participating in all sorts of activities, undertaking challenges and discovering new hobbies. The fear, which had spun an invisible web, slowly began to fragment and in its place the beginning of hope and anticipation began to glimmer. What was particularly formative was the opportunity to meet and chat informally with Robin Buttery. He lived and worked in the same city, was a father to a young child and was participating at the time in a scientific trial that involved rowing the Indian Ocean as part of a crew. In nothing more complex than sharing a couple of cups of coffee he raised the bar of possibility higher than I would ever have dared imagine or set it myself. This is the power of connection and the power of an individual. Just one person can make a huge difference. Since diagnosis, I have met with individuals who have cycled from

Land's End to John O'Groats, climbed mountains, started new companies and even written plays. Nothing enables or expands the possibilities of impairment more than connecting with those living with it and nothing will disable more than fear and isolation.

However, I was also very keen to connect with other healthcare professionals who were living and working with Parkinson's. I understood, very quickly, that the ability to maintain work was particularly important for me. There were several reasons why. Firstly, I love my job, and secondly, I'm someone who prefers to be active and busy. I have never relished sitting for long periods, and by the end of a two-week holiday on a sun lounger I am usually itching to get back to structure and routines. But as I began to talk things through, I discovered that work played an important contribution to the other roles of my life.

I think we often overlook the influence of culture and how it interfaces with our health. I grew up in Protestant Northern Ireland where a strong work ethos is engrained into every fabric of life. 'Work hard and strive to do your best in everything you undertake' was the motto of my upbringing. I learnt it at home, in school, in church and on the playing field. I was raised with the expectation to provide and in the belief that if you need or want something you work for it. That was the mindset of everyone around me and I never really questioned it, until confronted with the prospect of not being able to work. Then I became very aware of its influence on my thinking. I started to see that work formed an important pillar in my construct of a husband and father, that it was important to me that my kids grew up watching their dad work to provide for them. Yet diagnosed at forty-one years of age, with more than two decades of potential employment still ahead, I worried about how long I could realistically expect to sustain work. I understood the need to address some of my core beliefs in preparation for the future. I had to reframe work as a desire, an ideal and a goal, not as a necessity. That is less straightforward than it sounds and remains a work in progress.

My initial Google search for 'doctors with Parkinson's' didn't yield anything helpful, but with further searching, I stumbled across an article written by an obstetrics and gynecology physician in America called Dr Karen Jaffe. She was diagnosed with Parkinson's in 2008 at the age of forty-eight years and continued working until 2013. Although there were no articles about how she managed to practice medicine and work in healthcare with Parkinson's, I did read that she was seeing up to thirty-five patients a day and was continuing to deliver dozens of babies. However, what piqued my interest most was her decision to become involved in advocacy. She didn't go public with her diagnosis for three years as she feared stigma, a fear I could relate to (in the beginning I told only a select number of people at work), but five years after diagnosis she decided to close her practice and throw herself into this full time.

She became an ambassador for the Michael J. Fox Foundation's Fox Trial Finder, which helps to identify the right people with Parkinson's for the right trials, and she sits on the Fox Foundation's Patient Advisory Council. Furthermore, she became co-founder of a non-profit organisation which opened in 2015. This is a place where those with Parkinson's in her local area can learn how to live well. Various classes are made accessible, aimed at a holistic approach. The true value of this safe space was that people could find community with each other and discover the tools to empower themselves in the daily grind of what Parkinson's brings. She discovered that leading these exercise classes also acted as a great motivator for herself. Decisions to be open and public in your diagnosis are profoundly personal and there is no 'one size fits all,' but what I learnt is that my initial avoidance did not diminish fear and to the contrary enlarged it. I have never regretted the decision to start being more open about my illness. I found telling people lifted a burden off my shoulders and increased my support network. But I acknowledge that this, like so many aspects, is hard because it entails accepting some degree of vulnerability.

As I began to share my diagnosis and experienced the benefits of interacting with others, I was eager to do so as much as possible. Local support groups often met during the day when I was at work and I remained a little self-conscious, so I decided in the first instance to begin online. It afforded greater flexibility, and it felt less overwhelming to communicate from the security of my study. I had never engaged in social media before because I didn't have time or a particular reason to, but began to explore the familiar platforms of Facebook, Instagram and Twitter.

As a general trend I discovered colleagues tended to have Twitter/X as their professional social media profile and use Facebook and Instagram for their personal one. I wasn't drawn to Facebook as there was no limit to how many words I could type, and with Instagram I had to post a photo and I wasn't ready for that. So, I opted to open a Twitter account in 2018 with my name as my handle. I liked the challenge, and still do, of fitting what I want to say into one hundred and fifty characters or less, and I can choose to add a photo or video if I want. I soon found an active vibrant community online, as different as their symptoms but with one thing in common, everyone had been given a diagnosis of Parkinson's. Having made the decision to embrace being open about my illness I was also keen to get involved from a professional and personal point of view with Parkinson's within healthcare. This wasn't a huge step given my role in education, so when I was invited to speak at the Real Stories lunchtime series in Parkinson's UK headquarters in November 2018 I accepted. Addressing a lecture theatre full of students never fazed me, but after being diagnosed with Parkinson's my confidence seemed to vanish and though this was a small group the occasion provoked unusual levels of anxiety. Once again, I withdrew and turned down further invitations to speak.

The next time I spoke publicly about being diagnosed with Parkinson's was six months later at an evening organised in church, where I had an opportunity to share how my faith had impacted living with PD. Our church is a supportive community which feels like family and was therefore a very safe space. It helped assuage some of my anxiety for public speaking, and when I received an invitation to speak at the UK Clinical

Pharmacy Association annual conference in October 2019 I hesitantly agreed. This was the first opportunity to talk professionally about my experience of working in the ED with PD.

Travelling to Birmingham on the train the morning of the conference I could begin to see the early signs of adaptation. I arrived at the station car park in plenty of time, my phone was charged and I knew exactly where I was sitting. When the train pulled up, I let everyone else get on first, and before I entered my coach, I looked to see if everyone had sat down. I did the same when we reached New Street, waiting at the ticket barrier until it was less crowded. Progress often happens without awareness until one day the cumulative effects of silent adaptation in multiple increments becomes noticeable. This highlights another important principle of adaptation, faith. Just because you can't see change doesn't mean that it isn't happening. Roots must first be established before a shoot can sprout. It is important to be patient and to trust in the process.

A few months later I was invited to attend a Parkinson's UK Research Conference for the day. The Parkinson's Excellence Network (PEN) is the professional arm of Parkinson's UK, which brings together and helps health and social care professionals provide better support for people with Parkinson's and their families. In between the presentation of the awards, an NHS nurse, called Clare, talked about her experience of living with Parkinson's as a healthcare professional. I could relate to a lot of what she said about working in the NHS and living with Parkinson's. This represented an important first step in beginning to identify with other healthcare professionals. When we take a step forward we often do so without always understanding where the path will lead, but with the benefit of hindsight I can look back and recognise how these early opportunities acted as seeds that would sprout months, even years, later.

CHAPTER 10

Kyoto

As soon as I joined social media, I became aware how much the Parkinson's community extends internationally. Instrumental in broadening my horizons was discovery of an organisation called the World Parkinson's Congress (WPC), which since 2006 has held a conference every three years in different cities around the world. This conference is unique in involving the whole PD community. Neurologists, healthcare professionals, scientific researchers, people with Parkinson's and their carers can all attend together, at the same time. The next meeting was due to be held in Kyoto, Japan, in 2019, and although I thought it would be a brilliant conference to attend, travelling to Japan felt like a step too far. However, just as life throws up unexpected problems it can also bring unexpected opportunities.

Life is never as simple as clichés suggest and 'when one door shuts another opens' is a cliché. Being diagnosed with a progressive condition certainly closes some doors. Sometimes these doors shut because of fear, apathy, lack of education and grief, but difficult and testing circumstances can, if we choose to let them, bring new opportunities. When one door shuts it often enables a different one to be opened. The process of adaptation inevitably requires us to begin searching for open doors sometimes by pushing what seem like previously closed ones.

As a child I loved to draw. This interest had been sparked at the age of eight, when a family friend took time on a Sunday afternoon to show me how he drew illustrations. From then on, whenever it rained or I couldn't play football, I would spend hours copying cartoon characters from a picture in a comic or annual. Desperate Dan or Danger Mouse, it didn't matter, but Dennis the Menace was my favourite. Fifteen years later during a medical student placement on his surgical ward, the same friend said to me, 'Now I will teach you some surgery.' And he did exactly that using very clear drawings of anatomy on a whiteboard. For centuries art has been used to educate.

As a graduation present for Heather, I filled a sketch book with scenes from our time at university, and when Ben was a baby, I created cartoon characters of farm animals that were hung on the wall of his nursery, but it was years since I had completed a picture. However, one rainy lunchtime, around two years after diagnosis, I instinctively reached for the pencil on my desk and began to doodle on the napkin accompanying my meal-deal chicken sandwich. Ten minutes later I had completed a line sketch of a scene that had unfolded the evening before.

DOI: 10.1201/9781003600671-10

It was after dinner and I was sitting on the bottom stair attempting to tie my shoelaces and simultaneously finish a half-drunk, semi-warm cup of coffee. (It frequently feels like a taxi service in our house, with various clubs and groups throughout the week.) I was running late and Anna, who is a stickler for being on time, was fussing beside me. She was pressuring me out of the door, but I had forgotten my medication and being rushed caused me to become stressed. My anxiety levels rapidly escalated and, in the panic, I was unable to locate my keys. This would have been very uncharacteristic before PD but has since become a common occurrence. I have a small, cylindrical canister attached to them in which I keep my daily doses. I searched my right pocket, my left and then my coat which was hanging over the banister before finally hearing the jangle of the keys in the right pocket of my jeans where I had first started! I have noticed that when stressed I almost experience a perceptual blindness, failing to see things which are right in front of me. I cannot recall how many times I have spent twenty minutes frantically looking for something only for Heather to walk in and immediately point it out. By the time I took my medications out of the pocket I was so symptomatic I was unable to get the lid unscrewed. Anna, who had by now opened the front door, urged me on impatiently. 'Come on, Dad, we are going to be late!' But immediately after she spoke, she noticed my struggle. Closing the door, she took my keys and said, 'It's OK. We have time.'

Having completed the sketch in a simple line drawing, I returned to the business of ED but later that evening redrew it on an A5 piece of sketch paper, first in pencil and then in outline using a fine black ink pen. When finished, I scanned it onto my laptop and saved it in a file named 'Parkinson's drawings.'

Over the next few weeks, whenever I had opportunity, I reached for my pencil. I drew a picture of the queue to get through the ticket barrier at St Pancras train station in London. That was a real challenge as I had to get the details of the fabulous ironwork roof with its single arch. I also drew us all standing looking at the pavement to discover why I was tripping all the time. It is hard for me to sit in one place for any significant period but I discovered drawing helped me to focus and concentrate.

Each person was drawn with the first letter of their surname, so we were all A's. It's amazing how you can create characters from letters just by adding hands, feet and shoes that distinguish gender. The letters for the kids were smaller in size.

After I had completed ten drawings, I laid them on the dining room table rearranging them in the time order that they had happened. As I did so it became evident that they were becoming a means of telling the story of my diagnosis. I noticed that many of them captured those situations I had found embarrassing or upsetting.

For many, talking is a helpful way of processing emotions, but we aren't all the same. I don't find it especially easy to articulate what I'm feeling but I discovered that drawing was unexpectedly acting as therapy, helping me to work through challenging aspects of PD. I can't really explain but somehow the activity of drawing lines and constructing an image helped me process some of my frustrations. Perhaps it was as simple as taking something negative and, through the process of creativity, transforming it to something positive.

Weekends like evenings were always busy, and I recall one Saturday I must have been particularly symptomatic because I kept walking into the door frame. This happened a lot when I was tired. I didn't know whether I was misjudging the width of the door frame or if I was walking through it too quickly, but my shoulder would frequently collide with the wood, recoiling me backwards. On this day it had occurred several times. No one commented, but later that evening, when Anna was getting ready for bed, she went to the bathroom to brush her teeth and walked into the door frame 'Why did you do that?' I asked puzzled, 'To make you feel better,' she replied. It was a light bulb moment of realisation. This wasn't just therapy for me but could have broader applications. Anna had her own unique insight, and my drawings could be used to tell the story of PD through her nine-year-old eyes.

I drew twenty-six pictures in total and scanned them all into my computer before loading them onto iMovie. I wrote a simple script using scenes from the past two years of things that we had done together as a family and things that she had said and set it to music. When the WPC posted on social media that submissions were open for their video competition for the conference in Kyoto, I decided to submit it. The best twelve would be shortlisted and all would be shown in Kyoto. Once submitted to the WPC I nervously uploaded it onto YouTube and tweeted it out.

The reactions were wonderful to read and a real encouragement. A comment on YouTube read,

> This is a poignant and loving story from a child's eyes. Please enjoy and share. A diagnosis of Parkinson's disease is a whole family diagnosis. Everything will change but love remains, hope remains, and courage is pulled from deep within the young and old alike.

This was confirmation of the ability of art to also communicate and create emotional connections.

When we discovered that the video had reached the final twelve shortlist there was a decision to make. Travelling to a conference in Japan felt like a momentous step and a long distance to go for less than a week. I wasn't sure how jetlag would impact my symptoms or how I would manage my medications crossing international time zones, but I really wanted to see my video on the large screen. We also knew that it would afford us the opportunity to gain information on the latest advances and enable us to ask questions about areas we didn't really understand, such as the role of prebiotics. So, following lengthy discussion and with the help of Heather's parents to look after the children, we took the plunge and booked to fly from Birmingham to Amsterdam before transferring onto a thirteen-hour flight to Kyoto. (We knew nothing about Kyoto beyond that the 1992 Kyoto Protocol had been signed at an international United Nations conference which called for industrialised nations to significantly reduce their greenhouse gas emissions.)

To help plan our trip we bought a guidebook. Although we were only visiting for five days we wanted to experience as much of the local culture as possible. We would arrive around seven o'clock on Monday morning with time to sightsee before the opening ceremony on Tuesday evening. The conference would then run for three full days before we flew home on Saturday afternoon. I emailed my neurologist for advice on the timing of my medication. He suggested I take my medications as usual and advised that halfway through the flight to Kyoto, I reset my watch to the time zone in Japan and take further doses accordingly.

———————————

On 3 June 2019 we landed at Kansai International Airport, collected our bags and walked through the airport to the train station across the concourse. We bought a SIM card for our mobile phones and two tickets for the train which would take us from the airport to the centre of Kyoto in a journey of seventy-five minutes. As our departure time for the train approached more people arrived at the platform, but to our astonishment they lined up behind each other in an orderly queue. We were even more amazed when the train pulled in at the terminal and the seats on it rotated 180 degrees to face the opposite direction. It was a world away from St Pancras.

We had decided to stay at the hotel, just across the road from the International Conference Centre, as I wanted to preserve as much energy as possible. By the time we had checked into our hotel room I was desperate for the toilet, as is very common for people with PD. I had read in the guidebook about a Japanese toilet but wasn't prepared for what was about to happen. It looks like any other run-of-the-mill toilet, with a white seat, a white ceramic bowl and a small reservoir of water inside, but when you sit down there is a panel of buttons on the left. There are so many it looks like a TV remote. I have always been curious by nature, always ready to experiment so, out of interest, I decided to press them all. I went along the line slowly and carefully pressed one at a time waiting to see what happened. It was going well until I pressed the final button. The speed of the jet forced me to take a deep inhalation of breath. Wanting to stop it I looked back at the panel but couldn't remember which button I had pressed. I panicked and accidentally pressed it a second time initiating the jet once again and worsening my tremor. This time I stood up and automatically flushed the chain, deciding that this toilet had the same effect as working in an Emergency Department.

Travelling to Japan was a unique cultural experience and we had a wonderful two days of sightseeing before the conference started. Most of our anxieties about travelling proved unfounded. I coped well with the time change both regarding medications and energy levels. Heather and I have always loved travelling and when I was diagnosed, we thought it was something that would be restricted. But this trip to Japan was a great encouragement. We certainly had to adjust, limiting the itinerary, avoiding public transport in rush hour, arranging regular breaks and planning for toilet stops, but we almost didn't notice, and it felt good to be exploring somewhere new and doing what we loved.

During our breaks, we planned our time for the conference. The WPC scientific programme was forty pages long and packed full of options. In the top left-hand corner of the cover page were three phrases. The first was Advancing Science, underneath that was the second one, Promoting Community, and beneath that again was the third, Inspiring Hope. I knew I wouldn't leave the conference having advanced science, but I was certainly looking forward to meeting new people from the Parkinson's community and to being inspired about living with Parkinson's in the future.

Within the programme, there was a thermometer icon which graded the complexity of each talk. A green thermometer indicated that minimal scientific background would be required, a red temperature indicated a high level of scientific content, and yellow sat somewhere between the two. This was to assist delegates in their planning. The keynote plenary sessions were divided according to basic science, clinical science and comprehensive care, and twice every day there were roundtable and workshop sessions which allowed delegates to sit down with an expert in smaller groups. The overall aim of this unique event was for everyone to gain a better understanding of PD and to create a global dialogue that shared innovative science and best treatment practices and afford opportunities to work together in finding a cure for this complex disease.

The Grand Prize Video Winner was announced at the end of the opening ceremony. The winner was a filmmaker from Sweden called Anders M Leines. His film, *Keep Hope Alive*, was a wonderful tribute to Tom Isaacs, the founder of the Cure Parkinson's Trust (now Cure Parkinson's). He was yet another example of someone who wasn't content to settle for the status quo but had used his skills and experience to better the lives of those with PD, founding an organisation dedicated to advancing science in an effort to find a cure. As the announcement of the People's Choice Award approached, I leaned across to Heather and whispered, 'I may still have a chance.' 'No you don't,' she replied 'because you aren't sitting in the first two rows,' and so it proved. But in every way, I felt a winner because of this conference in Kyoto.

After the opening ceremony, as we wandered through the foyer, I began to recognise people whom I had connected with online. I met Larry Gifford and his wife Rebecca who were from Canada. Larry was diagnosed with Parkinson's in 2017 when he was forty-five years of age and had been in radio all his working life. He started a podcast called *When Life Gives You Parkinson's*, with the first episode being released in June 2018. He has since gone on to record six seasons, including one hundred and twenty-four episodes which have been listened to by more than four million people, and he uses his platform to educate, advocate and help others. When Larry and Rebecca started, only a few were recording podcasts, now there are many, but they set the bar.

It was so helpful and encouraging making these connections and I quickly determined that deciding to attend had been a great decision.

The WPC increased our understanding of Parkinson's together. The importance of high-intensity exercise was discussed many times. There were even table tennis tables at a room in the conference as well as interactive exercise sessions to give people a taster. We were also educated around the need to keep your speech and swallowing muscles strong. Losing my voice or choking was not something I wanted to happen. But above all Japan proved to be a special time because of all the people I met.

As I have already discussed, in the initial months after my diagnosis, I had largely chosen to avoid people with Parkinson's. But having overcome this reluctance I was now keen to meet as many people with PD as possible and learn from them. This conference helped me understand that my fear of the future and of getting worse had caused me to view those living with PD predominantly through the lens of their symptoms and in so doing I missed their individuality. As ED consultants we are trained to manage symptoms and therefore when we are reviewing and listening to patients that is our primary focus. But it can create a cognitive distortion which in turn generates an overly negative view of PD. However, in Kyoto, there were so many delegates with PD that at breakfast you certainly weren't the only person with a tremor nor were you the only person having to nip out during a session for a toilet break. This created a unique environment in which, for three days, symptoms became normalised, and the effect was that I stopped focusing on signs of disease. As I did so, I encountered wonderful stories of resilience, determination and accomplishment. During the conference, Larry recorded an edition of the podcast for each day. One of those interviewed was Matt Eagles, who was diagnosed with PD in 1975 when he was just seven years old. Although Parkinson's is more common in older people it can be diagnosed in children, when it is called juvenile Parkinson's. But it is extremely rare. Despite living with the condition for forty-eight years he continues to show and inspire how he has adapted to the condition. I will never forget watching him go down an escalator leaning forwards with bent knees and arms behind as if he was on a ski slope. It was priceless and made everyone around raise a smile.

A particular encouragement to me was to hear the account of one of the recipients of a special recognition award, Soania Mathur, a Canadian doctor who was diagnosed with Parkinson's at the age of twenty-seven and who worked as a family physician for a further twelve years after diagnosis. As she took the stage to talk about the physical and emotional challenges of living with PD for twenty years, it was clear that she was an educator. Her desire to advocate and empower those with PD to live well was inspirational.

Hearing stories and watching people with PD flourishing and embracing life acted as a real wake-up call. These people had not allowed PD to become the entire lens through which they viewed themselves but instead considered it as just one aspect of a bigger picture. They were patients but they were also campaigners determined to fight for 'better,' pioneers pushing boundaries, athletes setting new benchmarks, individuals redefining creativity, mums and husbands, colleagues and teammates. To see these individuals face PD head on – not denying the limitations but refusing to be defined by them – persevering with determination to use their experiences to help others advance education and promote care was so wonderful to see. I am indebted to their example and role in instilling confidence and for providing a vision of what life with PD can look like.

On the flight to Kyoto, I had checked my watch to discover we were less than halfway through the flight. It was one o'clock in the morning and there were another six and a half hours of flying time. As I wouldn't need any medications for five hours, I had reclined my seat and tried to get some rest. But after thirty minutes of fidgeting, I gave up. I looked over to Heather who was fast asleep and, not wanting to waken her, flicked through the movie choices and came upon the option of *Hacksaw Ridge*. This is a World War Two film about Desmond Doss, the first conscientious objector to be awarded the Medal of Honor for service beyond the call of duty, during the Battle of Okinawa in May 1945 in Japan. When the Japanese launched a huge counterattack many of the American soldiers were left injured on the battlefield, with the risk of being discovered by the Japanese and either killed or taken prisoner. What happened next was quite remarkable. When Desmond heard the distant cries of his comrades, he climbed up a sheer vertical cliff face on a rope, located them and carried them back to the cliff edge over his shoulder, before lowering them down to the ground, one at a time. In total, he lowered dozens of wounded and badly injured soldiers to the amazement of the rest of the unit below. The captain of the unit had a strategic plan to take the ridge the next day, which was a Sunday. But he would not execute it without Desmond present, so the assault was delayed until he had finished his Sunday prayers.

How we respond to adversity will be different for everyone, but what struck me in this film was Desmond's response when the lives of others depended on it. He didn't fight with his head, he fought with his heart and with what he believed in. He determined a course and when he faced obstacles, he demonstrated courage and bravery. Some people with Parkinson's like to consider themselves 'fighting' the disease. Others find the term unhelpful, but either way we can compare life with PD to the battlefield. We don't necessarily have to fight but we do need a strategy and, most importantly, like Desmond we need courage. Every day it requires courage to get up in the morning and venture into a world which has the capacity to hurl unexpected grenades. For many a trip to a restaurant requires bravery. Kyoto also helped me to recognise the role of courage in pushing against the natural drift of symptoms. I realised that as long as PD was seeking to slow and diminish my movements I had to counter – on the cross-trainer, the treadmill and bike – by pushing myself out of the comfort zone, but this is hard when you are afraid of falling and when you know that your balance and movements are not what they once were.

The WPC conference in Kyoto also lit within me a flame for advocacy, but the spark really belongs to the heroic individuals ahead of me whom I have watched navigate the battlefield with courage. In doing so they encouraged me more than they will ever know.

CHAPTER 11

Oz and Oil

The creativity that had prompted me to attend Kyoto was to develop further over the following months. I had witnessed at the conference how art can act as a powerful educator and given my interest and training in medical education it seemed logical to combine the two. However, my relationship with art has been complicated. Although I rediscovered a childhood love of drawing and had used drawings to illustrate Anna's story for the WPC conference, the truth was that in the three-month period, between late October 2018 and January 2019, I had drawn over one hundred pictures.

Six months prior to Japan, Liz, my Parkinson's specialist nurse, reduced my dopamine agonist patch from 10 mg to 8 mg and then by a further 2 mg three months later to 6 mg. She felt, after discussion with Heather, that drawing had developed into a compulsive behaviour and was being driven by the dopamine agonist. With the benefit of hindsight this course of action sounds more straightforward in principle than it was in practice.

Compulsive behaviours are simpler to recognise when they are new behaviours, out of character or causing obvious harm. When someone who carefully monitors their spending unexpectedly starts making multiple purchases online or credit is refused because accounts have gone into arrears, there will be little doubt about the existence of compulsive behaviour. When I was prescribed 12 mg of rotigotine it was very clear that I was experiencing compulsive behaviours in the form of hypersexuality. This was an unnatural, distressing feeling that was accompanied by agitation and anxiety when trying to suppress it. Drawing on the other hand was far more subtle and not as easily recognised as a compulsive behaviour. It was a hobby, and I was drawing before the agonist was started. I enjoyed it and was not experiencing any distress as a result. Indeed, to the contrary, drawing helped me feel relaxed and provided a sense of purpose. I used drawings to produce an Emergency Medicine Charity calendar raising money for Parkinson's UK and the Air Ambulance services locally and in Northern Ireland. I didn't consider my drawing compulsive and hadn't recognised when it progressed from adaptive to pathological. For Heather, however, it was a different story. She noticed the increase in intensity, the inability to spend a day without drawing and though I felt relaxed when I drew, she perceived the subtle shift that I was feeling agitated when I wasn't drawing. Whilst she was attempting to make dinner, run a taxi service and help with homework and I sat with my black pens and sketch pad, she did not find it helpful, and the reality was that for a period of several months, my drawing became a source of conflict. Usually, we work through issues together but on

DOI: 10.1201/9781003600671-11

this we were on different sides of the fence. I did not see what the problem was, and it took the objective input of Liz to help resolve the issue.

Living as a care partner of someone with PD is not always easy. When non-motor symptoms are pronounced it is as though the condition acts like one of those hoods used in racehorses to reduce the peripheral field of vision. It seems to create a narrow focus of perspective, generating blindness to the big picture and leading to fixed and rigid thinking. Conducting a rational argument on such occasions becomes untenable and has required us to change how we communicate. I cannot see the problem in the moment and Heather has learnt that no amount of conversation or arguing will persuade me to see what is patently obvious to her, the kids and everyone else. With time and improved understanding, we are learning to wait until there is better symptom control, such as after a dose, before completing a discussion. However, input from an objective voice can also prove effective at breaking deadlock. Ben, as he has grown up, sometimes acts as this voice but we have also valued the input from Liz. This is the importance of the multidisciplinary team and the benefit of continuity of care. She has taken time and skill over the years to establish relationships, building a broader, more holistic perspective beyond management of symptoms and medication. She understands our circumstances, the dynamics of the family unit and what normal looks like, and this enables her to be able to speak into situations when there is some form of complexity. We are very grateful for her expertise.

Sometimes it is easier for healthcare professionals to be heard in these situations than loved ones, and it is important that compulsive behaviours are carefully enquired about during reviews as they have the potential to cause significant harm to relationships. But caution is needed to ensure that the concept of impulse control is not too narrow. There is a risk of missing impulse control disorders when such behaviours develop out of pre-existing behaviour patterns. This is not an easy aspect of Parkinson's to manage. Diagnosis, as we have seen, can be difficult. There are no clear measures and so many variables which affect the picture. It is a very fine and distinctly blurred line between normal and abnormal behaviour. Perhaps the most helpful question to consider is whether a 'hobby' or activity can be temporarily stopped and put to the side for a break. If not, there may be benefit in exploring it further.

Once diagnosed the management can also be complex. The dose of an agonist can be reduced but this may cause a deterioration in motor and non-motor symptoms and so there is tension between symptom control and side effects which will be different for everyone. Furthermore, when the behaviour has been adaptive, it is not a simple case of discontinuing it. Something else needs to take its place. One option can be to introduce boundaries, but this too must be carefully balanced to avoid individuals feeling controlled. As the agonist was reduced and I adjusted to less medication I continued to draw but began to feel less agitated, and art became enjoyable once more.

After Kyoto, reaching the decision to use the medium of art to educate others was easy but I wondered how to accomplish it. Then, early one afternoon in August a message popped into my Twitter account from Parkinson's Europe. They had been at the WPC 2019 in Kyoto and were keen to discuss an art project. What transpired was a remit which perfectly fitted what I was seeking to achieve. They were redesigning their website to include a subsection describing symptoms, both motor and non-motor ones, and were keen to explore whether I could illustrate it.

The challenge was representing all the symptoms of Parkinson's artistically. My plan was to convey not only the nature and number of them, but somehow to embody what it felt like to live with each. I was especially keen to address those symptoms that I knew would be less familiar to the public. Many have written and spoken both descriptively and articulately on this subject, but my intention was to evoke feelings that would lead those observing to find out more. I wanted to get them thinking, contemplating and reflecting. Could I encapsulate in art what Parkinson's felt like?

The process developed easily. I drew the letters which spelt the symptom name and gave them hands and feet to create characters, hoping that those observing would consciously or subconsciously relate to them. Next, I framed them around a cartoon that visually depicted what the symptom felt like so people would feel drawn in and immersed in the picture. Finally, I added a short punchy strapline to tie it all together. These straplines described on a personal level the impact that symptom was having and how the individual with Parkinson's may have been feeling at that precise moment in time. Consider, for example, stiffness, a symptom felt acutely by many people with Parkinson's but one which is difficult to explain as it is unseen. Some present to a healthcare professional with a frozen shoulder as their first noticeable symptom and it can be years later before someone looks for and joins the dots realising that this is, in fact, Parkinson's. For me the joint that felt most stiff at diagnosis, and since, is my left wrist, often feeling like I need to give it a good shake to loosen it up. It's like an old window that hasn't been opened for a while and when you do it squeaks loudly at you, verbalising its resistance. When I am wearing off medications my left leg will also become stiff, feeling heavy like a lead weight. The speed and the mechanics of walking slow right down and when this happens, I always wish I could go into my garage, rummage on the shelves and locate a small can of oil that would make all the difference. A few drops on the bottom of the metal frame and the window moves easily and the squeaking disappears. How I wish I was like the Tin Man in *The Wizard of Oz* and could lubricate my wrist to make movement easier – so that is exactly what I decided to draw, obtaining basic supplies to get started in the form of a pencil, a rubber and an A5 sketch pad.

At the weekend I sat down at my study desk and carefully drew the word S-T-I-F-F-N-E-S-S on the A5 page, sketching it out in pencil first with my reliable eraser close by. I added the hands and a pair of little black boots to each letter and placed them all on a winding brick road. I drew separate squares onto the shape of each letter with small circles down two of the sides, giving the appearance of tin sheets that had been riveted into place. Each letter was completed by a cute little tin hat. The brick road background on which they were all standing was added with two wooden signs inserted at the bottom giving them the choice of which direction to go in. One pointed in the direction of Oz and the other in the direction of Oil with the strapline underneath that simply stated, 'I don't need Oz I need some Oil.'

In PD, unlike the film, there is no yellow brick road to be followed, no emerald city to be reached, no lion or scarecrow and certainly no Dorothy wearing a pair of shiny ruby shoes. Indeed, there often isn't a path to be seen at all. In the cartoon there are nine separate letters which could easily represent different individuals living with this condition, all on the same road but with individual experiences. But unlike the Tin Man, people with Parkinson's have a heart, plenty of heart, as they work out how to manage their symptoms. They aren't hollow but do have to learn to develop a steely outer layer that is protective, malleable and can withstand and cope with the stresses of everyday life.

Over the next six months, I drew a total of thirty-two cartoons in what I coined 'The Parkinson's Symptom Collection.' They included motor symptoms, non-motor symptoms and those which are side effects of treatment.

Shortly after they were finished, I had a chance conversation with the head of Arts and Heritage at the University Hospitals of Leicester, who had heard of my diagnosis. They are responsible for the upkeep of all the art within the hospital estate and were looking to put on a new exhibition near the main entrance. We got chatting about art, then about PD and finally about Parkinson's art and within thirty minutes a plan was hatched to launch the Parkinson's Portrayed Art exhibition. The next few months were busy as they were all printed on exhibition-grade paper and framed in slick black wooden frames. Underneath each was a description of the symptom being portrayed, as a key objective was to educate as many people as possible about Parkinson's.

All thirty-two frames were hung the day before opening with meticulous precision on the wall of a busy corridor. The estates team did a fabulous job in establishing perfect symmetry. With such a busy footfall along the corridor the exhibition provided a wonderful opportunity to not only educate healthcare staff but members of the public, so when it was confirmed that it would remain in place for three months, I was thrilled. Making a short thank you speech at the opening, I experienced an unexpected wave of emotion when I talked about the care of those with Parkinson's in hospital and particularly their difficulty in getting medication on time. This was the first time I had spoken publicly about Parkinson's from this perspective. Little did I know at that time that I would be working to get this issue on the national NHS agenda a few years later. The feedback from within the trust and from outside who viewed it when they were visiting was reassuringly positive, and some of the pictures were sold to raise money for Parkinson's charities.

The pictures were also displayed in the atrium of the medical school. Here exhibitions relating to health are installed for four weeks at a time by a local arts centre. Upon meeting them it was decided to have them reprinted on larger A3 paper given the height of the atrium but once again they were framed in black. It was fascinating to observe the response. I watched as medical students from first year right up to final year would come and look, read and educate themselves. At lunchtime, I would occasionally pop down from my office and ask them what they thought. It highlighted how few of them understood Parkinson's, and the lack of awareness of this condition amongst the medical professionals of the future spurred me on. As my artwork was installed in March 2020, I inadvertently hold the record for the longest-running exhibition in the history of the medical school, since it remained there until two weeks after the second lockdown ended. The destination and permanent home for all thirty-two of these pictures is now in the Neurology Outpatients Department. Before they were put up the whole area got a new coat of paint, including the doors, making it feel lighter and fresher. The drawings have also been exhibited in Belfast, Barcelona and Paris.

CHAPTER 12

Community

When Heather and I were married we had this verse printed on our wedding invitations: 'A cord of three strands is not easily broken.' We chose it to remind us that strength is found in unity, not in being unitary.

Community plays an important role in fostering well-being. Affirmation, challenge and encouragement need others to be present. Community can provide perspective, balance our weaknesses and offer support when we face what is fearful or unknown. If you are scaling a mountain and encounter a narrow ridge you must traverse it alone, but it will certainly be easier if you have watched others go before you and if there are encouraging voices behind.

I have already described how for the first few years I sought to manage PD alone. But in addition to this intentional avoidance there was also a slow creep of social withdrawal more generally. It was not that I was deliberately avoiding people, it was simply that it had become more effortful and as a result my participation in community had diminished.

It is important to acknowledge that PD can make relationships harder. I am a strong extrovert who relishes the company of others, but PD has impacted my social interactions in more ways than I sometimes like to admit. Since diagnosis I find it harder to sustain attention in conversations, which does not always make me a good listener. I am easily distracted, and my mind will often shift focus several times during a conversation so that I frequently miss what people have been saying. Furthermore, having lost the thread of conversation I panic and end up saying something completely tangential or irrelevant, making me seem both disinterested and odd. This is particularly the case in group gatherings where the possibility of distraction is greater. One of the earliest social adaptations we had to make was to limit entertaining to one other couple. Any more than this and I struggle. However, the problem also occurs over the breakfast table. Heather will be chatting and mention something that acts to remind me of a task at work or in the family admin that needs completing. I am immediately distracted and begin planning it in my head, meanwhile missing some important instruction or piece of information I'm expected to know at a later point!

Another frustrating manifestation of inattentiveness is the habit of interrupting. If I am listening to someone and think of something to say, I find it very difficult to

DOI: 10.1201/9781003600671-12

contain the thought long enough to enable them to finish their point. I'm so concerned about forgetting what I want to say before they have finished speaking that I have a compulsion to interject and talk over people, which can appear rude. Often, I'm not even conscious of doing so. Heather will give me a subtle nudge to let me know or catch my eye with a signal from across the room, but she isn't always present to do so.

Relationships are also hampered by loss of facial expressions. Non-verbal cues are an important part of communication and in PD we lose a whole dimension with masking. This is akin to switching facial expressions from colour to black and white and dramatically diminishes the range of emotions that can be expressed. I'm aware I can look bored, unmoved or detached even though I'm far from feeling it. This may be subtle but impedes the empathy necessary for deeper relationships, especially during conversations in which an emotional reaction would be anticipated by the other person.

Finally, when I am very fatigued and have a lot of non-motor symptomatology I can swing to the opposite extreme and exhibit a marked reduction in spontaneity of speech. There are days when Heather will highlight that although present physically, I have been totally detached emotionally. I may answer questions or directly respond but do not initiate any conversation, which is unhelpful especially if there are important family issues going on.

Kyoto helped me to see that I needed to be both proactive and intentional in re-engaging with community, even if it might sometimes be difficult. This was to become an important feature of adaptation. However, the first steps had already been embarked upon a few months earlier. Common ground acts as a great ice breaker and makes the hurdle of forming new social interactions easier. It feels safer to start with something we love and for me that was football.

The message on social media was short but immediately grabbed my attention. It simply asked anyone who was interested in being part of the UK's first Parkinson's football team to get in touch. The hope was to put together a team that would play in the Parkinson's European Cup 2019, a tournament held annually in Copenhagen. It will come as no surprise that the prospect of playing football in an international competition required little persuasion.

Ray Kennedy was an Arsenal and Liverpool professional footballer in the 1970s and 80s who was diagnosed with Parkinson's in 1984 at just thirty-three years of age. At the time he talked about the effect that it had on him and permitted his image to front a public campaign to raise awareness of the condition. The tournament was named in his honour and was the idea of Danish physiotherapists Finn Egeberg Nielson and Eigil Sabroe, who observed the benefits that playing football was having on their patients.

The UK Young Onset Parkinson's (UKYOPD) Football Team was formed online. We had never played together but had two things in common, a passion for football and a determination to live as best as we could with young onset Parkinson's. The team consisted of seven English players, Aaron, Barry, Charlie, John, Matt, Nick and Sam; three Welsh players, Ritchie, Roger and Garen; and finally me, from Northern Ireland. It was Sam's original idea to enter, Charlie put the team together and organised the logistics and Garen was responsible for the tactics.

A training day was organised for June so that everyone could meet for the first time. As we all lived in different parts of the country the most sensible place to hold it was Leicester. I booked an astroturf pitch and with the help of friends assembled an opposition team. It was a blisteringly hot day, so I filled the boot of my car with two-litre bottles of water to keep us all hydrated. Charlie distributed our sponsored kits – red socks, white tops and blue shorts: perfect colours for the UKYOPD team. The excitement mounted as we all realised this was no longer just a pipe dream and that we were soon to represent the UK at an international tournament. Despite the heat we made the most of the opportunity, discussing positions and strategy before playing the match. The final score was 8–6 to the opposition. We had lost but what mattered more was that we had bonded quickly as a group.

In July there was a further training session, this time with the first team at Morecambe Football Club when we were joined by a crew from BBC Five Live, a national radio station, to talk about the importance of exercise and Parkinson's. Not only were we benefitting individually from being part of a new community but we had created opportunity to change the public perception of PD. A few weeks later the team made an appearance on Soccer AM, a popular British football-based Saturday morning television show. In one of the regular segments, two teams compete in a penalty shoot-out. That day it was UKYOPD against a team of Nottingham Forest football fans. We won 4–3. Nick had placed his penalty perfectly in the corner, so we knew he was first on the team sheet if the situation arose.

The weekend of the tournament in September 2019 arrived at the end of a busy summer. Jules was joining me for support as part of friends and family, and as I waited for him to arrive, I completed a final mental checklist – medication, passport, boarding cards, shin pads and football boots.

Travelling with Parkinson's is always a challenge not just on the day of your journey but for a few days afterwards. When we had decided to take the kids to Florida in 2017, it was the first time after diagnosis that I had undertaken a long-haul flight across time zones. Uncertain of the impact on my symptoms and aware that I would be landing late in the evening and with disrupted medications, I had booked assisted travel. We arrived following a smooth flight and after landing were instructed to wait for everyone else to leave the plane. This was harder than it sounds with a seven-year-old who couldn't wait to meet Minnie Mouse. Once the last passenger had filed past, the cabin crew indicated that we could disembark but as I carefully descended the steps, I was aghast to discover an airport worker waiting to greet me with a wheelchair and not the motorised buggy I was expecting. I gave Heather a look that indicated my reluctance but after a short discussion where it became clear that it was this or no help at all, I sat down. As I was wheeled past queues and through the concourse to the baggage reclaim area I felt very conspicuous as though every pair of eyes were peering at me accusingly. They probably weren't but, in this situation, I was patently aware for the first time of the concept of hidden disability. I knew that I needed some help. I could feel the fatigue, the slowness and heaviness in my limbs after a 10-hour flight and understood that a lengthy walk and queuing were going to further add to the burden of my symptoms. But I also knew that I looked to all external appearances like a fit and healthy 43-year-old. Once again, my own pre-existing frameworks of disability were challenged and I was reminded that we shouldn't judge by what we see. As the alarm sounded and the baggage arrived on the carousel, my dismay increased further. I realised that I couldn't get out of the wheelchair to grab our suitcases, especially as our way had been cleared with loud announcement from the porter. Heather wasn't long recovered from a back prolapse and had to be careful lifting heavy bags so I was forced to watch helplessly while she and Ben grappled with the luggage. The whole experience left me feeling helpless and incapable.

I recognise the stage will arrive when it will be both necessary and helpful to have assisted travel, but I was determined to maximise my capabilities as long as possible. I needed a system that would recognise my difficulties and limit the impact of travel on my PD whilst facilitating my function and independence. It wasn't long after that I encountered the sunflower initiative. This is a free scheme in the UK that supports people with hidden disabilities and its discovery proved transformative. I had used it once before this trip to Copenhagen and it had been helpful, so when we arrived at the airport I attended the assisted travel desk to request one for the journey. It is very discreet and the staff didn't even ask why I needed it. I followed the sunflower signs in the terminal and was able to benefit from quicker check-in, fast-track security and priority boarding. This meant the queuing and standing time for the whole journey was reduced. It also helped reduce anxiety and the feeling of claustrophobia I experience in confined and crowded spaces. I continue to use it every time I travel, although some airports have moved to using a sticker system. It can also be used in some supermarkets and other modes of public transport. We have never flown without assistance or the sunflower symbol, so Ben and Anna are in for an awakening when they realise travel is not always so straightforward and that they will one day have to join the back of the queue! Unfortunately, it is not a universal system so sometimes it isn't recognised at the destination airport, but I have discovered that a conversation at check-in usually enables me to access whatever system is in place locally.

Upon landing in Copenhagen, Jules and I collected our bags and bought tickets for the train to the city centre, arriving in time to be able to check in to the hotel. We had a few hours to kill before dinner and decided to walk into the centre of Copenhagen to explore the 'Nyhavn,' an iconic sight in the city, with its colourful and captivating buildings all painted a different colour. Historically it was a commercial port where ships from all over the world would dock to conduct business, but today there is a mix of old boats and newer ones and most of the ground floors of these beautiful old buildings have been renovated into restaurants and pubs. When our coffees arrived at one of them, we sank back into our seats and enjoyed the sunshine. However, it wasn't the first time I had enjoyed this view.

'Do you want to come to Copenhagen in October?' my older brother, Peter had asked on the other end of the phone. 'I am trying to get tickets for the Denmark versus Northern Ireland game.' The two teams had been drawn together in the same qualifying group for the 2008 European Championships. My younger brother, Tim, had already confirmed he was free to travel and following a check of my rota I was soon on board.

I didn't do a lot of preparation as I knew Peter was extremely organised and would have every aspect of Copenhagen researched. And so, it proved. On the train he produced a travel file with train times and bus routes. It was a detailed degree of planning, but I was so impressed that ever since I have adopted the same practice. After dropping our bags at the hotel we headed in the direction of the centre. It was a warm October day, and the streets were filled with a mix of locals, tourists and football supporters, all enjoying the sunshine. Despite being from Northern Ireland, the fans who travel to away matches have earned the reputation of being amongst the best-behaved fans in the world of football. We had discussed beforehand what we wanted to see and looking at the map determined we were closest to the statue of Hans Christian Anderson. As we approached the Copenhagen City Hall Square we could spot the glimmer of bronze in the distance. The guidebook had described how the statue depicted Anderson sitting on a chair reading a book. But that afternoon he had become an honorary member of the Green and White Army (GAWA), draped in a green flag, with a green and white scarf tied around his neck and donning a large mad-hatter hat. He was having a busy afternoon with selfies. The square itself had been transformed for the day. A green haze filled the air, and the square was packed to the brim with fans, relaxing, unwinding and enjoying the atmosphere. There was talk of games in the past and the game that night, which was an important qualifier for the tournament being co-hosted by Austria and Switzerland. I wondered how we would get to the stadium when out of nowhere, a loud trumpet sounded that caught everyone's attention as it rang through the balmy evening air. It soon became apparent as the fans started to walk off the square in large numbers that the GAWA were on the move and were being given a police escort. We had no idea where we were going but just followed the throng.

In Northern Ireland when someone of older years addresses someone younger, they sometimes will use the word 'son' at the end of the sentence. The man beside me had been to every away game over the past twenty years. He was able to tell us that we were walking to the stadium. I didn't know where Denmark played their home games though was sure it would be bigger than Windsor Park in Belfast. We are walking to 'The Parken, son,' he said. I would look back in years to come and see the irony of that conversation. The trip remains one of those moments in life that are etched in your memory. We sang our hearts out and waved our flags and enjoyed an end-to-end game for ninety minutes. When the referee blew the final whistle at 0–0 the fans burst into song filling the Copenhagen with a rendition of 'Sweet Caroline.'

———————————

Eleven years later the streets were devoid of green flags and we weren't visiting the Parken Stadium, but the trip would be no less memorable. Football was the common thread but only so far in that it was acting to facilitate community. The benefit of relational connections would endure long after the whistle blew.

At dinner we met the other players who had arrived. Some had travelled with their wives and kids, others with friends, and there was a buzz of excitement, expectation and nervous energy. For the first time, we were united as a team and the excitement began to build even further. Charlie, our captain, gave a rousing speech at the end of the meal, summarising the journey over the preceding months. We had raised over £20,000 for charity and promoted the importance of high intensity exercise in Parkinson's across social media, radio and television.

The next morning we met for our first team talk. Garen explained the formation, before we gathered in the lobby to travel to the stadium. I wasn't sure what I was expecting but a very stylish coach appeared. We were all dressed in our team polo shirts and tracksuits and although we didn't know how we would play as a team, we at least looked like one. As I stepped on to the coach I'm not sure I would have felt any more excited if I was travelling to an FA Cup final at Wembley.

Arriving at the sports complex we registered, found our dressing room, changed and headed onto the pitches to warm up. It was a seven-a-side tournament with matches lasting fifteen minutes in total. We had been drawn in a group of four teams from Iceland and Sweden and our first opposition, Norway. The reigning champions, Stiff Legs, were on the other side of the draw so we wouldn't meet them before the semi-finals.

It was a hot day; the sky was blue and the sun was beating down intensely. We had brought plenty of water with us and slugged it down as all the players stood for a group photo. I stood with immense pride and sense of achievement as the president of the Danish Parkinson's Association talked about the history of the event, the sense of community and the importance of physical activity in living with Parkinson's.

Then the referee blew his whistle, and it was game on. The Norwegians were fit and fast and I was surprised at how big the pitches were for seven a side. It was a tense, tight affair and with only two minutes left on the clock it remained goalless. However as one of the Norwegian defenders attempted to launch a long ball to their centre forward, Matt intercepted, heading it back into the centre of the pitch whereupon I chested the bouncing ball down onto my left foot. I started running, acutely aware that two Norwegians were closing in either side of me. Protecting the ball I fended one of them off with my left arm but knew they were close to making a challenge. Spying the goal in the corner of my right eye, I spotted our centre forward, Charlie. As the defender extended to tackle, I passed the ball to him and he drilled it low and hard into the corner of the net. The referee blew his whistle. We had beaten the runners-up from last year 1–0, which wasn't bad for a team that had never played together. I watched as Aaron scored a brace in the first half of the second match and Garen knocked one in as well to help secure our second win against the Icelandic team. Ritchie, our goalkeeper, had made some brilliant reflex reaction saves to keep us in the match. Then we coasted past Sweden in our final group game 3–0. Roger, Nick, Sam and Barry had been solid in defence, and we had topped the group and reached the last four.

The semi-final was a cagey affair as most are. We had been drawn against another Icelandic team. They had one younger and very dangerous player who dictated and coordinated their play and they soon went 1–0 up midway through the first half. This was the first time we had gone behind in a match or conceded a goal in the whole tournament. They scored again with literally the last kick of the first half so we were 2–0 down at the break. When the referee blew his whistle to recommence the game, we had seven and a half minutes to score at least two goals.

We pushed like never before, and with three minutes left won a corner; I jogged over to take it. By now I was hurting but determined. Placing the ball down, I put my left arm up to signal that I was going long and following a short run-up, whipped the ball into the box. Matt had made a late surge forwards to score a diving header with one minute remaining. We had our heads in our hands when the referee blew the final whistle. We were out. It was a valiant effort, but we had come up short. Stiff Legs, the team from Denmark, progressed to win their fifth tournament, an impressive statistic.

After the games had finished it was time to have a meal together and to watch the presentation of the trophy. There was mutual respect for everyone who had taken part and a real sense of community. I was amazed by the effect of playing football. People who looked like they wouldn't be able to manage suddenly came alive.

As the speeches ended I grabbed the microphone and loudspeaker which were sitting beside me. 'Do you fancy singing a song? I asked Ritchie. 'What is it?' he replied. We googled 'Sweet Caroline,' opened it on YouTube, turned on the subtitles and started an impromptu sing-a-long. The lyrics took on a different meaning that day as we sang them. They could easily apply to Parkinson's and what we were trying to achieve.

Neuroplasticity is the term used to explain the brain's ability to form and reorganise new connections between neurons. I remember being fascinated when I first saw footage of a neuron trying to connect with another one, I was listening to music at the time and it was like watching a dancer, agile and nimble, stretching out, trying to touch the other. When we sang about hands reaching out and trying to touch other hands, I visualised my neurons doing the same. During the last chorus, all the players and their families joined hands and waved them in the air forming new connections. Back at the hotel, we sat in the courtyard and talked about the impact Parkinson's had on us all; it was cathartic.

Adaptation requires autonomy because it necessitates making choices, and the ability to choose is what defines our individuality. If change is imposed or compelled by others it is not adaptation in its truest sense. We aren't evolving as individuals but are being regulated and managed and there is an important distinction between the two. Management of progressive and degenerative conditions require elements of both adaptation and regulation in varying proportions depending on the stage. For example, medications, driving and risk are all regulated, but modifying lifestyle, making changes to our environment such as moving house or installing a wet room and requesting adjustments to work are all forms of adaptation. Illness can of course impair self-awareness and impact autonomy, but that is to venture into the separate territory of capacity.

Adapting requires an awareness of the need to change and acceptance that it is in our best interest. This is where the benefit of community can begin to emerge. Whilst community doesn't make the choice for individuals with capacity it can help inform awareness and guide individuals towards acceptance.

There is a country park we enjoy visiting with the kids and one section has an area of naturally built obstacles and challenges designed to test balance and coordination: wooden beams, climbing poles and frames. We have been visiting it for years and each time my competitive instinct surfaces in determination to prove to myself. I can still complete them just as well as ever. Of course, success depends on when I last took my medication. If a dose is due then my symptoms can frustrate the process. Heather will stand observing as I refuse to move on until I've managed each one, despite an evident worsening of my symptoms, enquiring whether it really matters and pointing out it's 'just as important to notice the birdsong and enjoy the walk!' But however much she may reason, in the end I must choose between continuing to persist, tiring myself in the process, and further depleting my dopamine or accepting that on this occasion I can't manage it, quietening my determination to instead enjoy time with the family.

Community manifests in various forms. I could as easily talk about the role of my extended family, the support of church members and of course the team I work with. So many avenues of life guide us towards community: faith, work, hobbies, volunteering and neighbourhood. I consider myself very fortunate to benefit from a variety of interlinked support circles, each one contributing something unique to ensure I am well supported. Family provides love, challenge and safety; my PD groups inspiration, understanding and encouragement; my faith assurance, rest and hope; my work perspective and purpose; and my friends laughter and normality. This has not happened overnight but taken time to develop and frequently requires effort and perseverance. I have also learnt lessons on the way. It can be easy with PD to become blinkered and overly focused on one thing to the detriment of the big picture, and much like exercising only one muscle this can create imbalance. There have been periods when I have needed to pull back from one aspect of community to spend more time in another.

Community will unsurprisingly look different for everyone. There are no set rules or formulae and it doesn't matter what community looks like. It may be the baristas in the local coffee shop, the trainers in the gym, a key worker or healthcare professional, the neighbour who pops in to see if you need anything from the corner shop or an individual whom you've met virtually in a community forum about bird watching.

I also acknowledge that it can be much harder for some to achieve than others. Those who struggle significantly with anxiety and apathy can end up isolated, and it is important for health and social structures to be proactive in supporting and enabling individuals to take steps that may feel overwhelming and frightening in the first instance, but which potentially could bring them great gains in the longer term.

A Weeble was a roly-poly children's toy in the 1970s with a weight that stopped it from being pushed over, and for me that is exactly how my support team function. When at times things get too much or I am heading too far to one extreme, they are there to prevent me from falling over or act as a counterbalance to help me rediscover equilibrium.

CHAPTER 13

COVID

When I arrived at the counter there was a mutual nod which indicated that one regular latte was on its way. I never needed to order from the hospital cafe as I drank the same coffee every morning. As I pulled a chair out to sit down at an empty table the Emergency Department Head of Service came to join me. Although Vivek was my boss, he was also my friend. We had both started in the ED on the same day in 2004, progressing together through specialist training and exams to our eventual appointment as consultants.

This morning the mood was subdued, reflecting the atmosphere which had permeated every department of the hospital. Even in the canteen, where there was normally a symphony of conversation, voices were quiet, and it was impossible to escape the sense of nervous tension. Aware of the growing pressure on his time and workload, I took the opportunity to garner his opinion and asked, 'What do you think I should do?'

It was March 2020. COVID had arrived on British shores and the healthcare community was preparing for the unknown. The UK government had just released a list of health conditions which put people at higher risk of complications from COVID and Parkinson's was on it. I had studied the early evidence describing the devastation COVID was wreaking on the fit and healthy, not to mention the clinically vulnerable, and was therefore very anxious about the possibility of contracting it. However, I was also conscious of the pressures which were about to face my colleagues. ED is a team and in the moment of crisis when the metaphorical 'frontline' was about to become a real one I wanted to be there, alongside everyone else, playing my part. It felt like having been trained for battle but, when war was eventually declared, asking to be relieved from duty. It didn't sit comfortably, and I felt torn between fear and guilt. This was the second time I had asked this question of a healthcare professional (the first being immediately after diagnosis) and it reflected the level of perplexity I was feeling.

Before diagnosis I would have listed decisiveness as a personal strength. I was typically someone who could evaluate options, weigh up the pros and cons and select a course with relative ease and speed. But that is no longer always the case. Determining what to do, particularly when decisions are emotively charged and have important implications for the family, demands more time, and it is effortful to avoid becoming stuck in a pattern of overthinking. On each occasion I have needed to alter my pattern of working, I have felt like a hamster running over the same ground again and again, before being able to settle on the right course of action. The uncertainty makes me

DOI: 10.1201/9781003600671-13

feel very anxious and I end up paradoxically resisting the impulse to make a snap decision simply to obtain symptomatic relief. This triad of symptoms – impulsivity, indecisiveness and anxiety – are inter-connected and often augment each other with anxiety leading to indecisiveness and impulsivity and vice versa. It can be complex determining which is the root problem. Interestingly indecision is most evident at either end of the spectrum of consequence, in those decisions which have huge personal impact and those which have no real significance at all. I have noticed that my symptoms are frequently worse on a Sunday compared to other days. It's the time in the week when we tend as a family to relax and be less task oriented, and I think I might miss the natural dopamine release that accompanies ticking boxes on a list. Perhaps it is just the business and tiredness of the week catching up as I slow down, but either way Heather and I now have a running joke that we can determine how the day will unfold by how many times I have changed my outfit before leaving for church.

Decision making is a complex cognitive function associated in the literature with many areas of the brain. One such region is the prefrontal cortex located in the front part of the brain. This region has an important role in what is collectively termed executive function. As the name suggests this is the 'managerial' level of brain function which organises, coordinates and integrates other aspects. Several non-motor symptoms in PD are associated with dopamine depletion in these frontal circuits. However, as symptoms they can be elusive, unpredictable and vague in nature, making them especially challenging to manage. It requires a double-edged approach, involving proactive measures to limit their occurrence in the first place and reactive measures to respond when they do.

We live with open countryside at the back of our garden. Rats are an ever-present reality, but they usually remain on the far side of the fence, and we can ignore them. However, we are never sure when they might surface as unwelcome guests. We have measures in place to limit this likelihood; we don't hang bird food, have pruned back shrubs to create open space and created an edging of stones so we can detect burrowing. But we also have traps on hand for those times we spot a disappearing tail. In a similar manner cognitive non-motor symptoms are a daily reality which largely remain in the background. However, there are periods when they 'cross the garden fence' to become troublesome and make their presence felt.

Improved knowledge and the benefit of learned experience has enabled me to implement preventative measures by anticipating situations likely to impact symptom control. I know that failure to maintain my exercise routine worsens non-motor symptoms, so I ensure I have access to a gym when we book a hotel. If I have attended a conference or meeting far from home, I choose to stay over rather than travel late in the evening and we plan flights for holidays in the morning. I time coffee and lunch breaks when my dopamine levels are low so I am cognitively resting and we try to ensure important decision making for the family is planned and undertaken in the morning when I am medicated, the house is quiet and there are fewer demands on my attention. Recently Heather helped me organise my wardrobe. Clothes are all on hangers tied with different coloured ribbons, blue for work clothes, red for casual and so on, so I can more easily determine what I am going to wear. Such measures appear minor and inconsequential but over the course of a day and week they operate cumulatively to reduce the overall burden of decision making, conserve dopamine and diminish the burden of non-motor symptoms.

Establishing routines is also beneficial for symptom management. Thursday is my morning off and we have a favourite coffee shop where we sit at the same table with the same order. This may appear rigid but it is not. I am never annoyed if the table we sit at is occupied and we do frequent other coffee shops. This is adaptation brought about through considered choices and prioritisation. Such routines, which necessitate minimal decision making, conserve my dopamine for what is important such as the ability to concentrate on what we will discuss over coffee!

However, there are periods when despite every best effort I still find the way forward hampered by indecision. This is the occasion to bring out the traps, the time for reactive measures, and the best one, I have ascertained, is to seek help and advice from someone you trust. Today there has been a considered shift away from the paternalism which frequently characterised medical consultations in the past. And this is a good thing. It is imperative that the principles of consent are fully upheld and that autonomy and decision making remain with the patient unless they lack capacity. But as doctors I think we often forget that even when we are ill, we operate from an advantageous base. We have knowledge, we have easy access to good quality evidence-based information and we have friends and colleagues we can discuss things with informally in helping us reach decisions. But not everyone has this benefit, and even with it I have been surprised how often I have sat in a consultation, having my questions answered, listening to information to discover by the end that the single question I most want answered is 'What do you think?' When we feel vulnerable and confused there resides within us all a desire to be guided. In most situations this can be met outside the consultation room but for some, those who are isolated with little support or without the ability to navigate their way past medical language, this is not always so easy.

Vivek and I had a discussion and agreed that I would work from home for the immediate future. On reflection this was the right decision. At this stage, no one knew what we were dealing with or how severe the impact would be, and we considered it best to err on the side of caution. However, I did not relish the prospect of working from home and COVID was to prove a challenge from both a physical and a mental perspective. I had worked hard to establish an exercise routine but now the gym was closed and I needed to find alternative ways of maintaining activity. One of my colleagues kindly gave me a Turbo trainer which could be attached to my road bike, allowing me to continue cycling in my garage. At 6.30 am, four times a week during the first lockdown, I got on my bike and cycled for thirty minutes. Breakfast and my stretching routine followed before opening my laptop to see which Teams, Zoom or Google Meet calls awaited that day. My NHS work continued Monday, Wednesday and Thursday, the medical school Tuesday and Fridays.

My concerns that there would be insufficient work for me to complete from home were quickly dispelled. In the early days of pandemic planning, it became clear that if the worst-case models were to play out a rapid expansion of the workforce would be needed. Legislation was passed to facilitate those with training to return to practice under emergency relicensing, and a request was made to all medical schools to expedite the graduation of final year medical students. This posed a huge challenge. We had a cohort of senior students who were only three months away from graduation but they had not been formally assessed, and to ensure public safety and validate their degree this would be essential.

It normally takes a team a year to plan and organise final examinations, but this time, for practical purposes, all assessment would have to be undertaken online and there was no precedent for that. We had to develop three, twelve-station exams from scratch and to raise the stakes there was a tight deadline of four weeks. I lost count in the end how many hours it took to re-plan the circuits, write and edit stations. We were unable to have any clinical examination, practical procedures or simulation stations as they couldn't be assessed over a screen and had to instead concentrate on stations involving history taking, communication and interpretation of investigation. There was a whole new acronym invented during COVID – the Modified Online Clinical Assessment (MOCA). Once the thirty-six stations were finalised, actors and examiners required training on the logistics of how this virtual exam would run.

The pressure mounted daily as the date of the exam approached. The potential for error was huge. If a student failed to enter a station online and on time during their allocated slot it would cause chaos for the running order. We had to include additional 'blank stations' in case any student encountered technical problems or for any reason a station needed repeating. Finally, we had to establish communication channels via a WhatsApp group between the administration team, the senior examiners and markers to deal with unforeseen circumstances.

I was on tenterhooks as examiners began to enter the Zoom examiner briefing, at eight o'clock on the morning of the first day. With a minute to go the administration team messaged to confirm everyone had arrived. That had never happened before in our face-to-face examiner briefing as someone always arrived late. Thankfully in lockdown there were no school runs to do or car parking spaces to find and it augured well. The same happened for the next two days and although some students didn't manage to technically enter some of their stations on time, this was identified early and they sat them at the end of the circuit. A huge advantage of conducting the assessment online was that each station was recorded so if issues arose whereby the student felt disadvantaged, we could review the footage as it had happened in real time. Overall the MOCA ran smoothly across the three days, with minimal incident, which was a credit to the whole team, examiners and students.

These two months highlighted the importance of cognitive flexibility. I had to respond to change with little warning and throughout this period was not able to follow pre-existing protocols or procedures, nor practise within conventional and established frameworks. I had led a team through uncharted waters without maps to follow and demonstrated that although I had to contend with non-motor symptoms, I was still capable of creativity, innovation and implementing novel ways of working. It was enormously encouraging and enabled me to reframe my approach to work. Since diagnosis my focus of thinking had perniciously and progressively centred on what had diminished, on those things I found difficult or could no longer accomplish, and the effect had been a gradual erosion of confidence and self-esteem. COVID helped redress the balance and shift it back towards those things I can do and do well. I acknowledge limitations still exist but recognise that so too do possibilities. Fear in all its forms acts as one of the greatest barriers to quality of life. I could spend every day peering through the window watching in case rats appear or I can put measures in place, do what I can and get on with it until a problem occurs. This empowers me to manage my PD rather than permitting it to manage me. The shift is subtle but is one that enables adaptation rather than imposing disability. As I described in an earlier chapter, I am definitely not able to undertake the extreme end of rapid decision making necessary in resus and majors, but I am fortunate that there is still a lot of work in the ED which occurs at a lower intensity of pace.

I also began to approach the management of PD in much the same way I manage a shopping budget. COVID had demonstrated what was possible. For an eight-week period during lockdown I had sustained a particularly high intensity of cognitive work, in part facilitated by reduced demand in other aspects of life. I found I was able to make more dopamine available for cognitive work because I wasn't driving and so on. I realised that in the same way that you can't afford to drink champagne or eat steak every night you could budget them in occasionally by cutting back somewhere else. I can plan in days which I know will be extra demanding if I am willing to tolerate subsequent days where my symptoms may be noticeably worse and I may be able to manage less than usual. This again is helpful in generating a small locus of control in a condition which is difficult to regulate or predict.

After three months of working upstairs out of a box bedroom I was desperate to return to work. I missed clinical practice and seeing patients and was acutely aware of the pressure the department was under. I had seen pictures on the news and read how my colleagues were coping through our WhatsApp group chat and hospital emails. I understood there was risk but I wanted to help. Although I still wouldn't be able to work in the main ED, with the right personal protective equipment (PPE) it was decided I could return and work in EDU, which would free up one of my colleagues to go back to the main ED bolstering the numbers there.

I distinctly remember feeling nervous driving to work on that first day back, but there was also a sense of relief walking through the main entrance. The corridors were empty except for occasional staff members hurrying to where they needed to be and it reminded me more of the atmosphere in the hospital at three o'clock in the morning than at the start of a busy day. My colleagues looked tired and strained. It was incredibly warm to wear PPE for a whole shift especially in resus and it was difficult to keep hydrated. I completed my PPE training session and by the time I walked into EDU and started my ward round later that day I was itching to get going. It felt good to be back practising medicine, part of a team and making a difference to the lives of patients.

EDU remained busy. Even though the country was in lockdown emergencies continued unabated. I remember seeing a patient who had been admitted on a mental health pathway having taken a drug overdose. Her bloods tests were all within the normal range and she had been admitted for observation to ensure the medication she had taken in excess didn't cause any delayed symptoms. Although her heart rate was slightly high when she first arrived, this had settled, and all her observations continued to be normal. I explained to her that the overdose had not caused any harm and that I was going to refer her to the mental health team to see what support they could give her. When I asked if she had any questions she immediately replied. 'Do you know why I look like an 'Oompa Loompa?' I have been asked many questions during my career but I wasn't expecting that one. I looked at the junior doctors in my team that morning who, even through their masks, looked puzzled. I glanced at the EDU nurse who shrugged to confirm she was as mystified as me. It was plain to see her skin was definitely an orange colour. We pushed her bed into the corridor to inspect in natural light but it still appeared orange. The EDU nurse explained she had assumed the patient was simply wearing false tan. But the patient shook her head and replied, 'It's not.'

Jaundice can cause the skin to appear yellow, a low blood count causes it to be pale and certain drugs can cause it to turn a blue-grey colour when exposed to sunlight, but I had never seen skin that had gone orange before. I went back to basics and asked a few more questions. 'Has this happened before?' 'No' she replied. 'What medication are you on?' I enquired. 'I don't take anything,' she answered. Medicine is also about observation, and although we all had assumed her orange tinted skin was false tan, I looked around the bedside and I noticed a fitness magazine on her cabinet. 'Do you exercise a lot?' She nodded. 'I have signed up to a few online exercise classes during lockdown,' she added. 'Do you follow a specific eating regime with your exercise programme?' I asked. 'Not really,' she replied, 'but I have been eating more vegetables recently, especially carrots.' That was the clue that would give the answer to this diagnostic dilemma. 'How many carrots do you eat a day?' I asked. 'Most days about ten to twelve, I have been doing that for a few weeks as I am a trying to lose some lockdown weight.' She had a condition called carotenemia which is caused by eating too many carrots. Carrots contain beta-carotenes, which if accumulated in the body can turn the skin orange. It wasn't harmful and it would disappear when she reduced her intake of carrots. She couldn't quite believe it when I told her.

In an earlier chapter I considered the phenomenon of muscle memory where repeated and rehearsed patterns of activity remain possible even in the presence of significant motor dysfunction. In a similar manner in which I can lift a skipping rope and rotate my wrist, I find decision making in work has remained much less affected than at home in part because of the repetitive and honed nature of it. I have been making clinical decisions for many years and am well practised in what I am doing. My knowledge base has been cultivated over three decades and because I operate with the benefit of objectivity, emotion impacts decision making to a lesser extent that in the family.

Work during the first lockdown proved to be an important milestone and reassured me that I was still able to add value despite the challenges of living with Parkinson's. Adjustments were necessary and though symptoms occasionally make work more effortful I can still use my training, communicate with patients, make observations and identify verbal and non-verbal cues.

COVID was another seismic event and a time of national adaptation. All the normal structures and routines of private and public life changed suddenly. There wasn't one response needed but multiple. However, what it demonstrated is that when change is forced upon us, we can adapt. It may not be easy, we may not like it, but we eventually find a way to establish a 'new normal.'

COVID reassured me, beyond the parameters of PD, that I can not only adapt to new situations but in so doing discover alternative ways of finding joy in life. Consequently, I am now less fearful of change. I would obviously prefer for things to alter on my terms, but I accept that they won't. However, what I also comprehend is that I have the capability if I choose to use it.

Change is ultimately driven by hope. When we find our backs against the wall, stuck in the mud, it is conviction that there is something better beyond our current circumstances that ultimately propels us forwards. Hope is essential in the process of adaptability, which is why despair and depression must be resolutely managed in enabling those living with progressive conditions.

CHAPTER 14

Compromise

To sail a boat requires skill to change tack and read the direction of the wind. The skipper is constantly reviewing the conditions, the sail positions and the nautical speed to ensure progress. Adapting to symptoms which are variable and constantly changing requires similar appraisal to determine whether modifications made have been effective or indeed detrimental. For this reason, incorporating regular periods of review is an integral part of the adaptation process. In March 2020, I reached a crossroads in the medical management of my Parkinson's, in part because I was increasingly experiencing the phenomenon of 'wearing off.'

I don't know anyone with PD who enjoys the sensation that occurs when medication prescribed becomes less effective and breakthrough symptoms develop between doses. When I first started Stanek each dose would last six hours. I would administer it at six o'clock in the morning, midday and six o'clock in the evening and notice few, if any, symptoms in between. But, over time the efficacy of this dosing schedule diminished and my periods of 'wearing off' lengthened.

'Wearing off' can be experienced as motor symptoms, non-motor symptoms or a combination of the two. I have both but their impact is different. My motor symptoms cause my left arm to stiffen and my left leg to feel heavy like it's strapped to a tonne weight, but although it is uncomfortable I remain mobile. Indeed, rather than slowing I begin to observe a tendency towards increased motor activity. Heather characterises these episodes as the 'Duracell bunny.' During them I walk faster, occasionally stumbling in my haste. I become unable to sit still for even five minutes and cannot settle on any activity until eventually Heather intervenes to insist I stay in one place for at least ten minutes knowing that when I succeed and eventually manage to stop, I will inevitably be asleep in the chair within five minutes.

My non-motor symptoms are more variable, as I have alluded to, but often I develop pronounced fatigue. The term 'brain fog' is widely used in many different contexts. I'm not sure what this means for others, but I can relate to the sensation of losing mental clarity and experiencing disorientation. It is as though someone has injected water into my brain. Such non-motor symptoms impact my function and as I have highlighted are considerably more disabling than the motor symptoms are. Furthermore, because they are invisible, they are more difficult for others to identify. When you break a bone and are wearing a cast, people can see that and respond appropriately. Perhaps wearing a sunflower lanyard in the workplace would be a way

DOI: 10.1201/9781003600671-14

of saying, 'I don't want to make a big deal about this but at this moment in time I may need a little more support.'

Over time such symptoms breaking through between doses were managed by adjusting either the dose or the timing of my medications. However, by this stage in March 2020 my neurologist was reluctant to increase my levodopa beyond the five doses of the red Stanek tablets I was already prescribed, as he considered this would be more likely to cause dyskinesia.

PD is the result of damage to neural circuits leading to loss of dopaminergic cells. However, the pattern of damage is not uniform. Characteristically in PD, the movement pathways in a region of the brain known as the substantia nigra are prominently affected. Low levels of the neurotransmitter dopamine give rise to the classical symptoms of slowness of movement, stiffness and tremor. The purpose of levodopa is to augment these low dopamine levels thereby reducing motor symptoms. However, levodopa is far more like a carpet bomb than a targeted missile. There is presently no way of being able to direct it only to pathways which have been damaged. Instead, it has the effect of increasing dopamine in all parts of the brain, creating imbalance in unaffected pathways and leading to symptoms which are the result of excessive dopamine. Dyskinesia is considered an example of one such side effect.

In Kyoto I had witnessed people with Parkinson's with disabling dyskinesia. They weren't in control of the movement of their bodies as their faces grimaced or their arms and hands twisted in a writhing, even rhythmic, type of movement. Aside from the psychological impact, this contributes to fatigue and weight loss as the constant motor movement throughout the day increases the body's metabolic needs. It can be a troublesome side effect and so for the first time I was conscious of a tension between a desire for more levodopa and better symptom control and the risk of introducing new symptoms as side effect. It was a tension that was not easily resolved.

Medical management almost always involves some trade-off between symptom control and side effects. This can vary from individual to individual and is influenced by several different factors.

The first are patient factors, those which are specific to the individual. Consideration is given to body mass index (BMI), allergies, other health problems and medication history. We have already considered how my strong family history of alcohol dependence influenced the decision to prescribe dopamine agonists.

Secondly, the decision depends on context. In ED the context is usually acute, often involving emergency and critical scenarios. Whilst we are always mindful of side effects the balance of decision making is usually very much weighted towards symptom control because the consequences of failing to treat the symptoms far outweigh the consequences of side effects in the short term. For example on EDU we prescribe Oramorph (a liquid-based morphine medication) for patients with acute back pain which isn't controlled by oral painkillers. This can cause them to feel very nauseated and cause them to vomit. However, this usually settles after a few doses. They tolerate the side effect because without it their pain wouldn't be as well controlled. If that nausea were to continue then the balance of decision making would shift.

Another influential factor affecting the balance of decision making is the degree to which treatment impacts survival or function. Where management significantly alters either of these then balance almost always shifts towards favouring treatment and tolerating side effects. In PD management this relates more to function than survival, but assessment of this tends to be subjective which raises its own problems. Traditionally the phenomenon of 'wearing off' Parkinson's medications is assessed predominantly in terms of motor symptoms. They are easier to measure in terms of function, can be assessed objectively and communicated more effectively and are less affected by other variables. When you attend a clinic review it is easier to explain that when your dose is due you become unable to manage stairs or that you scuff your foot more frequently. Non-motor symptoms on the other hand are frequently overlooked by both patients and clinicians. There are several reasons why. Firstly, without education many patients do not recognise their indecisiveness or diminished ability to conceptualise as a symptom of executive dysfunction and therefore are less likely to report it. Secondly, most clinicians have significantly less training and experience in assessing cognitive function than physical examination and are therefore more confident evaluating motor symptoms. Finally, as doctors we tend to focus on assessing what we treat and at present we medicate according to motor symptoms, and yet for me non-motor symptoms fluctuate much more than my motor ones and cause far more impairment of my function.

Decision making is also influenced by clinician factors. In medicine, learning is not just acquired knowledge, it is also acquired experience. It involves developing your own system based on what the evidence shows but also on what you observe and learn in practise, throughout your career. An adverse reaction may be very rare but if you have directly encountered it in clinical practice then it will inevitably influence your future prescription. All neurologists have access to the same drugs to increase the levels of dopamine but how they choose to prescribe them differs, depending in part on patient factors. In some cases, particular medications may not be prescribed at all and there may be different upper limit of doses, timings and combinations, but even accounting for this there is still variability between clinicians. This is the art of medicine. Healthcare professionals are constantly adapting and evolving their practice, and there are differing opinions. It is especially true in the management of syndromes where the pathology is not clearly understood and where the purpose of treatment is not disease modification but symptom management. Where medications are being prescribed to modify a specific and measurable factor – consider the use of statins to reduce cholesterol, insulin to reduce HBA1c or inhalers to improve peak flow – then prescribing decisions tend to be more straightforward. Presently, management of PD is based on subjective clinical observation and subjective patient experience rather than objective disease markers. There is a large diversity in presentation and many variables impacting symptoms such as physical health and mobility. Because of this it can be difficult to establish the evidence base necessary to produce approved and standardised treatments. Whilst the evidence base is growing all the time there is still not always a clear consensus. As a patient this can be hard to navigate. It can feel lonely and isolating because there is no clear comparative, and when you listen to others with the condition they can seem to be heading in the opposite direction. My patient journey has felt more like following a track through countryside that occasionally disappears than a concrete, well signposted path. There are points when I have needed to stop, to try and identify some marker that will help gauge the right way forward. This is not travelling on a motorway where, once you are on the correct road, cruise control can be activated; it is driving through unfamiliar terrain, in sometimes foggy weather. It requires active engagement and participation in the process. This engagement is time consuming, anxiety provoking and involves a lot of executive function – the very thing patients with PD struggle with. It is especially difficult for those who don't understand the landscape or know the markers to look for. We have considered how there has been a welcome shift away from paternalism towards actively involving patients in their treatment decisions. However, it is worth remembering that to make truly informed decisions patients need to be presented with all the facts and evidence in a manner that can be understood, which is the reason high-quality information to educate is crucial.

March 2020 was a time for appraisal – a point where I needed to stop, survey and take stock. With reflection up until this point I had operated with an unconscious bias towards aggressive management of symptom control probably because of my ED training. My tendency was to give greater weight to the immediate and short term with much less consideration of the longer-term picture. With hindsight I can recognise that I had a low threshold for reporting symptoms as impactful and tended to assess my response to medication and overall function far more in quantitative terms than in qualitative ones. In short, I considered treatment success as being symptom free rather than symptom controlled.

My neurologist at this time shared the belief that early and aggressive management was the best way to maintain function in the longer term, and the result was that my medications were titrated up quickly. This helped to maintain excellent function and control of symptoms but within three years and by the age of forty-five I was beginning to run out of road regarding medication options. The neurologist was reluctant to increase my oral levodopa tablets for the reasons I have outlined and his preferred management was to refer me to a neurosurgeon for a consultation about the possibility and suitability of undergoing deep brain stimulation (DBS). This would enable me to reduce the dose of levodopa, lessening the possibility of dyskinesia.

However, DBS is not without risks. This is a surgical procedure which is carried out in two stages. In the first stage, fine electrodes are placed in a specific area of the brain by drilling two holes in your skull and placing them in a precise area to the exact millimetre. It is performed when you are awake, under local anaesthetic, so the surgeons can monitor any change in your voice or movement. The second stage is performed under a general anaesthetic where a pacemaker is implanted in a pocket in the chest wall and connected to the wires that have previously been tunnelled under the skin from the skull to the chest wall.

There is no local neurosurgical service in Leicester, so one crisp spring morning Heather and I dropped the kids to school and took an early train sixty miles north to Sheffield where we discussed the pros and cons of DBS with the neurosurgeon. His overall recommendation was that he would be willing to progress and arrange the assessments necessary for DBS to take place but his personal opinion was that it would be equally valid and reasoned to delay. Given the lack of clear consensus, we decided to defer a decision for six months.

This period was very stressful. I just didn't know what to do and this was a big decision. Furthermore, it would be fair to say that this was a rare point where Heather and I digressed. In addition to symptoms and side effects, medical management of PD must also balance the short-term and long-term picture. PD is a progressive condition but typically does not significantly shorten survival. There are a limited number of drugs with limited doses, few other treatment options and no imminent cure on the horizon, so management options must be considered over the potential lifespan of the patient. The younger the age of onset the more this becomes a consideration. Heather, as a psychiatrist, has more experience managing chronic conditions and had a different perspective. Unlike me she gives more weight to the long-term picture. She was concerned that my expectations were unrealistic, that I was focusing too much on the short term and that I may regret having a lack of options further down the track. She was concerned I was not willing to make any compromises to PD and that whilst I was functioning well I was still existing in a degree of denial which was influencing my decision making.

I felt that I needed more information and so we discussed the issue with Liz. To help reach a decision my GP also referred me to another movement disorder neurologist for a second opinion in September 2020. It had to be on Zoom due to lockdown restrictions. He suggested a different levodopa tablet which if I took it at six in the morning would last longer to perhaps four o'clock in the afternoon, as it was released into my body at a slower rate. This would help to smooth out any wearing off. I would still feel the effects in the evening, but my day's work would have been completed by then. I felt reassured by the plan and was relieved when it provided better control.

In the end after numerous discussions and much advice I decided not to proceed with DBS, as Heather and I both agreed the benefits at that stage did not outweigh the risks. I was still maintaining a very high level of function and although my symptoms affected the quality of my function they were not regularly impacting it quantitatively.

It was at this juncture I learnt another critical component of adaptability – the need to accept compromise. Until this point, I had not truly grasped this. If I am honest I hated having any symptoms and my tolerance of them was very low. It didn't comfort me (when it should have) that I was able to do everything I wanted. Instead, I was frustrated that I couldn't do it as well or as quickly as I desired, and there is a subtle difference between the two. The former results in gratitude, the latter leads to discontentment from where it is very hard to find acceptance. I was trying to reach the point where my symptoms were so diminished in the background that I could continue living almost self-forgetful of my diagnosis. But I had to accept that these expectations of medical management were idealistic rather than realistic. Perfect symptom control in PD is an illusionary aspiration because of the progressive nature of the condition and the limitations of the treatment options currently available. Hopefully the emerging development of levodopa pumps and infusions will improve this soon, but presently the choice is not deciding whether to accept a trade-off but in determining which one you make. This represents yet another very personal decision that will be different for everyone and influenced by many factors including age and symptom profile. Both our kids were still young when I was diagnosed, so by titrating levodopa early and delaying DBS, I accepted an earlier risk of developing dyskinesia to maximise symptom control and maintain function as much as possible through their childhood and to continue working in the ED. But others will make different choices. However, the dynamic nature of PD and our personal circumstances mean that these evaluations are never fixed and must be subject to review. I do not use the same parameters to reach decisions today as I did five or six years ago. I continue to dislike experiencing any symptoms but I have evolved to accept a certain level as part of my everyday experience. Rather than focusing on the ten to twenty percent of my motor function that is impaired, I consider instead the eighty to ninety percent that remains intact. I now also only tend to become conscious of symptoms when for whatever reason they reduce my function well below my new accepted baseline. This has normalised some of my impairment and enabled me to begin to accept some compromises and to further the process of adaptation rather than remaining stuck in denial. It was to prove an important evolution when, in the incoming months, I would face some hefty compromises.

CHAPTER 15

More Symptoms

In September 2020, I decided to stop working at the medical school as the lead for clinical assessment. I had been preparing OSCEs for nine years and the truth is that after designing, writing, planning and running the MOCA during COVID my heart just wasn't in it. I felt burnt out. I had sat down in August to begin preparation for the next year's exam and couldn't find the motivation or creativity to write the stations. I was also beginning to struggle coordinating two separate workstreams at the medical school and in the ED. The ability to shift between tasks, to leave one set of jobs unfinished and to pick up work on an entirely different set, is yet another aspect of executive function which can be impacted in PD. Since diagnosis I have become increasingly aware of an inability to leave tasks unfinished. I much prefer to complete one job before moving to the next than to have lots of plates spinning simultaneously, and once I start a task, even if another of higher priority presents itself, I am reluctant to leave the original until it is complete. However, life does not always operate according to a timetabled agenda, especially when you have children. The unexpected happens; schedules may be written in a diary but frequently alter; tasks are reprioritised and sometimes everything must be set aside to respond to an emotional crisis. None of this is easy with the symptoms of PD, which prefer predictable, planned and repetitive routines and calm, stable environments.

My struggle at that time was due to an especially significant burden of non-motor symptoms, and I was beginning to develop symptoms of both low mood and apathy, which were new for me. The change was driven in large measure by inadequate sleep.

I have always been someone who enjoyed good sleep, but PD has certainly altered my sleep architecture. Since diagnosis it is unusual to hear the high-pitched beeps of my phone alarm set for 5.45 am, I am always awake well before this. An early start means that in the evening I watch the clock with drooping eyelids from 8.30 pm onwards. If I sit in front of the TV I will frequently drift into slumber, and by ten o'clock I am usually headed to bed. It is not uncommon to waken through the night for the toilet, but there is never difficulty in falling back to sleep. However, in mid-2020 this suddenly changed. I would fall asleep as usual, but almost as though injected by a shot of caffeine I started waking at 2 am, bright and alert. From then it was relentless tossing and turning. If I was fortunate, I fell asleep at three, only to reawaken at four. With a quiet house and everyone else in deep slumber, time marched slowly, prolonging the hours. The instant the digital display hit 5.00 am, I crept out of bed to end the torture, whether there were signs of early morning light or not.

DOI: 10.1201/9781003600671-15

After a poor night's sleep, I was always more symptomatic, which is no surprise given the amount of dopamine I used up tossing and turning. The unremitting nature of the problem meant that over time the cumulative effect was a significant worsening of non-motor symptoms. Nothing I tried helped. Although I only drank decaffeinated coffee, I didn't have a cup after 2 pm. I avoided screen time for an hour before I went to bed and I didn't read when I got there. We put darkeners on the curtains and we turned the heat down in the bedroom. I put in earplugs, wore an eye mask and even tried melatonin, all to no avail. Nothing worked. To make matters worse my restlessness began interrupting Heather's sleep and having both of us exhausted was a recipe for discord, especially as she has chronic migraines triggered by lack of sleep. We talked about what we should do. We discussed the option of a bigger bed but decided Heather wasn't Goldilocks. The spare room was an option, but we felt that once this decision was made it would be hard to reverse. In the end we visited a store and learned we could buy a bed where both the mattress and base could be split and separated if needed. That hasn't turned out to be necessary, but we discovered the change to two separate mattresses, zipped into a king, has made an enormous difference. If I am restless there is not as much transmission of movement and Heather's sleep is less disturbed.

Mum also suggested using a natural remedy that she had been recommended which she ordered for me from a high street shop. But within three days of starting, I noticed an abrupt and significant worsening of symptoms. It felt as though my medications were not working at all. I had horrible stiffness down my left side, and my foot felt as though it had transformed to lead. We felt the coincidence was too great to ignore and after persisting a few more days I discontinued them. Within 48 hours my symptoms had returned to baseline. There was nothing in the ingredient list to suggest there should have been a problem, nothing known to interact with my medication, but it was a timely reminder of the importance of not assuming that just because something is herbal or natural it won't have an adverse effect. It also reinforced the importance as a clinician of enquiring about over-the-counter medications and of the need to advise those individuals keen to explore natural remedies about the need to be vigilant. Because of the degree of impact I had experienced I submitted a yellow card to the Medicines and Healthcare products Regulatory Agency (MHRA). However, their response indicated that because it was classified as a food supplement and not a medicinal product they were unable to follow it up. They did helpfully suggest referring it to the Food Standards Agency to investigate and after contacting the supplier who conducted an internal investigation it was concluded there was no potential source within the product that could have made my symptoms worse. It remains an enigma. However, what is not a mystery is another interaction that I had experienced a year earlier.

Drug interactions are common, and it is well documented which medications should be avoided in people with Parkinson's, but healthcare staff will occasionally still prescribe them unknowingly. A fungal infection had developed and worsened in my left big toe, and following an appointment with my GP I was prescribed oral terbinafine tablets which I took as directed (treatment is long term for several months). A few weeks later I was sitting in the medical school writing an OSCE when I observed a pungent smell of burning oil. The nature and degree of the smell was intrusive and distracting me from my work, but I was unable to locate the source. It persisted later at home and I began to wonder if it was somehow emanating from me. It was beginning to cause agitation, but Heather could smell nothing. However, when I complained about it several times the next day, she quickly recognised that it was an olfactory hallucination.

I considered how levodopa is indiscriminate in its ability to alter dopamine levels in all areas of the brain, whether affected by PD or not, and that in some instances excessive levels can give rise to symptoms. Hallucinations, like dyskinesia, are considered one such symptom. A quick check in the drug formulary confirmed that terbinafine could interact with rasagiline, potentially increasing its effect. This increase had caused hallucinations. I immediately discontinued it and although it continued for a few more weeks it eventually settled and has never returned. Alternative antifungal medication was prescribed. Ever since I am very careful to check and read every word of the small print of any new medication and check for interactions.

Because of the burden of non-motor symptoms at this point, Heather and I both considered that something had to change to sustain my long-term ability to work, and I had a difficult choice to make between my two workstreams. It involved weeks of deliberation because of a quandary which is common in the management of all chronic and progressive conditions. I wasn't sure if my symptoms at the time represented a permanent change and were indicative of a new baseline or whether they represented a period of natural fluctuation with potential to improve. We had no crystal ball and, in that moment, had to make the best judgement possible, given the evidence in front of us.

I loved the work in both the ED and medical school but they each also had their own challenges. In the end the decision came down to two things: firstly confidence but most influentially the people. I have worked in six different EDs during my career. They have all been busy and stressful but in each of them, without question, the highlight has been the sense of community and teamwork, and by the team I mean everyone – from the managers, nurses and healthcare assistants to the admin staff security team and porters. When things get busy there is a real sense of 'We are all in this together,' everyone playing their small part, each as important as the other, all working hard to achieve the same goal of helping the sick. In my first weeks working in A&E I can still recall being in resus one afternoon when a patient was admitted unconscious with a partially obstructed airway, the air coming out was noisy as if he was snoring. It resolved if I manually lifted his jaw forwards but I couldn't hold that forever so I turned to Brigid, the A&E nurse, 'I need a . . . .' But before I had completed my sentence to ask for a Guedel airway – a plastic piece of equipment that is inserted into the mouth to protect and keep the airway open – she was beside me, already waiting to hand it to me. They come in different colours which represent different sizes. 'I think a green one will be the correct size,' she said. So, I measured it, and she was right.

When I felt at sea after my diagnosis, the whole ED team were a lifeboat, and those who have played a central role know who they are. I am so thankful for their input and support and can categorically assert I would not still be working nine years later if it was not for their help. This book is about enabling patients to live well. I was extremely fortunate to work in a team and for a trust who have done that every step of the way, accommodating adjustments and displaying flexibility. I had confidence this group of people had my back and although when I was first diagnosed I had believed my work in ED would stop before the university in the end, I didn't want to lose this community.

However, relinquishing my title of associate professor in medical education was not easy. I had worked so hard to earn it and felt I had barely got my teeth in the role before it was gone. For some time, I felt sad and despondent. I have heard people use the phrase, 'Parkinson's is the disease that always takes away.' I don't know that I fully agree with this as there are many positive things that PD has given to me, but in the moment that I shut the door on my office in the medical school for the last time, those words never felt truer. However, I was proud of what I had achieved over nine years, half of them while living with Parkinson's, and the assessment process was in a healthy position.

Time and hindsight eventually provide answers. It was indeed a prolonged fluctuation and the symptoms did eventually settle, and perhaps I could have continued with both jobs for longer. I will never know but it highlights another important aspect of adaptability. We may not get every decision right but backward glances will just fix us to a spot. The only way to move forward is to keep looking ahead.

The two days I had been working in medical education were transferred to the hospital so I remained full time. I continued EDU ward rounds, but these were changed to Monday and Tuesday and on those days, I also answered all the complaints, investigated any incidents where a patient may have come to harm and provided the trust with an ED opinion of a case that had come through to the legal team. This work suited my Parkinson's well. It is task driven with multiple boxes to be ticked in a day and the ability to complete the list and start each week with a largely clean slate. It keeps me focused and helps my concentration. I was enjoying clinical work again but there was one symptom that persisted, and that was my ongoing lack of sleep but with an added dimension.

I had believed my issues with dopamine agonists were behind me but in March 2021 I developed the side effect of daytime sleepiness. I was experiencing this especially around lunchtime and into the afternoon. On a Wednesday afternoon, I ran a medical education teaching clinic where junior doctors could bring an ED case that they had seen and discuss it with me as part of their training. Week after week when they started to talk about their patient, I could feel my eyes glaze over and began to feel very sleepy. I just couldn't keep my eyes open. It reached a point where my head would drop down towards my chin quickly and then jolt back upwards. It was embarrassing and I began to become very aware of it impacting my life. It would happen in meetings if I was not directly engaged or was sitting for a prolonged period not speaking. I had also noticed that when I was sitting in the car's passenger seat the sound of the engine would also cause me to drop off. Though there had been no problem I began to worry that it would affect my ability to drive, and we decided that I should not drive until I had spoken with my consultant and found a resolution. In total I chose to cease driving for five months until my levels of fatigue had improved and the episodes of sleepiness stopped. This felt like yet more compromise but in the loss, there was unexpected gain. Heather dropped me into work and picked me up again and we had an extra hour of quality time without distractions to chat and in the end, I missed it when I returned to driving. It also highlights an important point that change isn't always permanent and sometimes we can reverse compromises.

I didn't have another appointment for several months so I emailed my neurologist who wrote to my GP suggesting a further reduction in my dopamine agonist patch in April 2021 from 6 mg to 4 mg. The advantage was that the patch was becoming progressively smaller so I had more space on my arms to locate one in a different place every day, avoiding irritation of my skin. At the next neurology review my consultant suggested the introduction of amitriptyline, a medication to help with my sleep which would also have the added benefit of stopping me from getting up in the middle of the night to go to the toilet – another non-motor symptom that was not helping with sleep or fatigue! After the first dose, I woke to a noise that I hadn't heard in years. Rousing from a deep slumber I reached across and turned my alarm clock off. I had slept all night. As I walked to the bathroom, the sun was shining and the birds were singing. That simple introduction was transformative. I continue to waken routinely every morning around 5.20 am but overall I sleep well and obtain a regular seven hours each night.

A few months later I began experiencing episodes of dizziness when I stood up from a chair or bent down to pick something off the floor. My eyes would glaze over for a second as my body adjusted to what was happening. I felt as if I was about to pass out. I tried standing up slowly but that didn't help. After it had repeatedly happened in work, I booked myself in to my own ED to be assessed. About forty-five minutes later a care of the elderly consultant came to see me. Like being in a wheelchair this felt uncomfortable, but our neurology services are based at another hospital in the city and the reality was he was the doctor with most experience of managing people with Parkinson's. He was very thorough listening to my symptoms, examining me for any clinical signs that may give a clue to what the cause was. He checked my bloods, and my blood pressure lying and standing. These were all normal as was my CT head scan. He explained that although my blood pressure didn't drop when I stood up he felt that there was an imbalance in the system that controlled it. 'Do you drink caffeinated coffee?' he asked. I shook my head as I had given up caffeinated coffee a few years prior to diagnosis. He advised that I should restart having a maximum of two cups a day with the last one not being after four o'clock so it would not disrupt my newly established sleep. Within a few days the symptoms resolved. Again, something simple had brought about a dramatic effect, however I am learning that Parkinson's is always a balancing act and no more so when there are two symptoms in tension with each other. Although the caffeine helped my dizziness it also sensitised my bladder and I found that no matter where I was an hour after drinking a cup, I needed a toilet urgently. I have even had to download an app on my phone that tells me where the nearest toilet is if I am out in town and I recently ordered a Radar key.

Towards the end of 2021 the symptom I had been seeking to avoid began to emerge. I noticed it for the first time one evening watching a Champions League football match with Ben. My left foot began to move involuntarily when it was crossed over my right foot. It would move from side to side, round and round, up and down in no pattern and was exacerbated by stressful situations. I also noticed that when I was concentrating on typing a complaint response in work, if the front of my left foot was planted on the floor the rest of my foot would start involuntarily moving my leg to the edge of the table. Over time it has progressed to affect my torso, causing me to writhe forwards and backwards in my seat. As it has worsened it has begun to have more of an impact. It is certainly tiring – I am wearing shoes out more quickly and have noticed a need to increase my calorie intake to avoid losing weight. However, the most difficult aspect is the awareness that others notice. For so long I have lived with PD and though I have felt it, the external manifestation has been subtle and difficult to spot except when I am wearing off medications. But it is becoming increasingly obvious, even when other symptoms are well controlled, that I am living with a neurological disease. And so, I have entered a new process of adaptation and am working through the impact.

I have reflected many times if I had to do it all again would I follow the same treatment path? My medications were titrated up quickly and it did take a lot of medication to get my left arm swinging again. I had a bumpy ride with finding the right combination of medications at the right dose causing a lot of personal difficulty, but I would not change the quality of function I enjoyed through the critical years of family life which enabled me to enjoy so many experiences with the children.

It is important to review and reflect. It is often helpful to look behind to see how far we have come but what I have discovered to be unhelpful is to retrace old steps, and that is what regret does. It is like coming across a junction on a woodland trail and taking a turn that loops you back round what you have just walked. It consumes unnecessary energy and stalls progress. Regrets hinder adaptation.

CHAPTER 16

Healthcare Professionals with Parkinson's

Anyone diagnosed with a chronic condition acquires a new dimension to their identity and there are several ways of managing this. The first is to put your head in the sand, try to pretend it's not there and plough on as normal. A second option is to keep it separate from other aspects of life but that is difficult to do. However, I discovered there is a third option, integration. This shifts PD from being something that happens to you to becoming one part of the bigger picture of who you are. This is adaptation that moves beyond acceptance to transformation, but it isn't easy. It requires patience and there is no set formula to be followed.

Everything changed in an instant the day I was diagnosed and yet for a long time it felt as though nothing had. It was a period of metamorphosis. I was no longer who I was before but hadn't yet discovered how to embrace who I am now. For the first few years I was cocooned, all my energy absorbed by the process of transition. It wasn't a period of passivity but a time of intense learning. Learning to manage my symptoms, learning to understand the illness, learning new routines, learning to be vulnerable and adjusting to limitations until I eventually discovered a new normal. Of course, the reality with any progressive condition is that any 'new normal' is never permanent, but there are plateaus when life stabilises and when managing the diagnosis no longer consumes every ounce of your energy.

For much of the first three years I had been operating in the mode of compartmentalisation. Several factors were instrumental in shifting me towards integration. I began to see that PD gave me an additional perspective as a doctor and vice versa. My faith framed PD as something that could be used for good to serve others, and I had begun to see that being a patient informed my role as an educator. As I started to make these connections the horizons of possibility immediately expanded. Rather than being separate parts of a whole, my art and job and love for education, my desire to improve the lives of others, my physical health and my faith could all be linked and fused together. I'm not a psychologist but this for me was integration, and what emerged from the melting pot was not something I had foreseen at the time of diagnosis.

Football had connected me with people with Parkinson's on a personal basis and set in motion a new course, but something was still missing and that was a connection with people living and working with Parkinson's within the NHS. Seeds of advocacy, sown when reading about the work of Karen Jaffe, began to take root and my desire to connect with other healthcare professionals was re-ignited.

DOI: 10.1201/9781003600671-16

I had been working in the NHS for long enough to understand how slow and difficult the process of change can be. When I had first started as a consultant in ED, I was tasked with the responsibility of overseeing the resus equipment drawers. As part of that role, I wanted to implement a simple redesign and introduce dividers within them. It took two years and numerous meetings to succeed in doing so. I immediately recognised that alone I would make minimal impact. However, if I could mobilise a group of like-minded individuals then together there would be possibility to achieve so much more.

Kyoto had provided opportunity to meet another NHS nurse and a doctor living with Parkinson's. That amounted to three healthcare professionals whom I knew of in the UK, but I was certain there had to be more. I just didn't know where they were or whether they wanted to be found and if I did find them what we would do as a group.

Towards the end of the first COVID lockdown I contacted Clare Addison, whose story I had heard at the Parkinson's Excellence Network Research Conference in 2018, and floated the idea of starting up a virtual Parkinson's support group for healthcare professionals who were working in the NHS and living with the condition. At this point the primary aim was support.

PD varies from individual to individual with everyone experiencing a different mix of symptoms that appear at different ages and stages. Despite this everyone seems to be put into the same Parkinson's book, when in fact we might be not on the same page or even in the same chapter. In any condition where there is such large diversity it is easy to feel quite isolated because it can be difficult to locate those who can relate to your experience of the condition. This is why forming groups simply based on PD as common ground isn't always effective. An alternative approach is to base them on some other common ground such as football or singing or in this case occupation. This means even if my experience of PD in relation to symptoms is different, my experience of working with it in the NHS is similar, and this facilitates the connection necessary for relationships to develop.

In August 2020 during the first COVID lockdown, we formed the NHS Professionals Living and Working with Parkinson's Group to help support each other. We sent out a tweet asking for Medical Twitter to help us find other healthcare professionals who had found themselves in a similar situation. Within twenty-four hours there were eleven of us. I couldn't believe it, we had a paramedic, two radiographers, four nurses and three other doctors. We set up a WhatsApp group with a few ground rules: no posts before seven o'clock in the morning and none after eight o'clock in the evening. We decided initially to restrict the discussion to a Thursday and centre it on a question that one of the group members would pose in turn. The individual nominated would ask a question which could be related to Parkinson's or not. We also decided to have a Zoom meeting once a month which was open mic; a chance to discuss and talk and support each other. There was a two-week break over Christmas and at Easter and six weeks in the summer. A few weeks after we started, I recalled that Nick, whom

I had met playing football in Copenhagen, also worked in the NHS. I contacted him and invited him to the group. We now had an NHS manager, and there were twelve members in total.

At first the group was established for individuals presently working in the NHS, but we quickly changed to include those who had previously been working in healthcare but had now retired. They needed support too as they transitioned to living with PD. Two retired GPs and a nurse joined. One had made the voluntary decision to retire early after they were diagnosed. The others had gone through the process of ill health retirement.

In January 2021 we decided to make a short film, and everyone could choose to opt in or out of the project. Ten of us volunteered. First, we needed a structure that a script could be added to. The idea was floated that we should focus on working in the NHS and highlight how we felt at diagnosis regarding whether we would be able to continue working. We wanted to convey a feeling of self-belief but also reassurance to show our family, friends, work colleagues and managers how we could still work with Parkinson's with adjustments in place. Finally, we wanted to blend how incredibly proud and thankful we all were to work in the NHS with the stark realism that over time our lives and our work would change as our Parkinson's progressed.

After a few weeks of writing, editing and tweaking we agreed on the words and the format. It would consist of two sections. In the first part, we all would speak to the camera directly on four separate occasions. To begin with, we would state our name. This would then be followed with our age, our job title and finally how long we all had been living with Parkinson's. The second part would pose the question, 'What does it feel like to work in healthcare and live with Parkinson's?' This section required two separate recordings, one video clip of us either in our NHS workplaces or working from home and the second a voice recording of the script so that the narrated words would voice over the video footage. I forwarded instructions for people to record their footage in landscape with the person doing the recording holding their phone or tablet horizontally. As this was during COVID we all had to be wearing facemasks if we were to be filmed in clinical areas. We also had to gain consent from all the NHS trusts where people were working before the cameras could start to roll. Once the film portion was complete, everyone then recorded their narrated words.

After all the footage was gathered, I began the process of editing. The biggest challenge was adjusting the volume as some people had been closer to their phones when they recorded their section. The music was chosen and at the end we added a blank screen of text that simply read, 'Dedicated to all who look after us, motivate and encourage. Their care enables us to keep caring.' Finally, we collectively agreed on a title, 'Connecting through Care: The Inside Job.'

The completed project was uploaded onto YouTube and posted on social media on the 11 April 2021, which was World Parkinson's Day. It was watched by families, friends, work colleagues and our employers, giving them a little insight into what work meant to each of us as we adapted to life with PD. It showed everyone that we still had the passion and drive to provide good quality of care. More importantly it demonstrated the increased potential in working collaboratively.

The group grew steadily in numbers over the next few years, mainly through word of mouth and social media. Over time healthcare professionals began to get in touch with us and to pass on our details to others who they thought might benefit. It was clear that the group was a safe space, and it has become a great pillar of support. We continue to expand and as of January 2025 we welcomed our fiftieth member.

Naturally, the group dynamic has changed the bigger we have grown, but we have maintained our original structure with the nominated Thursday question still being a great source of information and discussion alongside the online meetings. Over the years three questions from a Thursday have stood out. The first one was, 'How has Parkinson's impacted your relationships?' This was a far-reaching question. Usually when the question is posted the replies follow quickly, but not this time. It wasn't until the afternoon that the first post appeared reflecting the complexity of the issue. People were honest and open, and it proved very helpful. The second was, 'What has made you really smile and be thankful this year?' I liked this because it made us all look outwards and not inwards and helped us to take stock and appreciate the small and sometimes overlooked things in life that bring us joy. The last one was, 'If the group was to make a Spotify playlist what song would you include?' By Friday morning we had a brand-new playlist that people could listen to while they were exercising.

In 2022 we felt as a group that we wanted to raise awareness of the diversity of PD and decided to make another short film. Again, this was split into two sections. In the first, we each stated the symptom that was most difficult to live with, and in the second, we explained why. What transpired illustrated the variety of Parkinson's symptoms. Amongst the ten of us who took part, everyone said something different.

Anil explained that anxiety was one of the main non-motor symptoms of his Parkinson's and that he found that episodes of his anxiety increased the frequency, speed and amplitude of his hand tremors, which were quite disabling. Sally described bradykinesia and explained how in her role as a practice nurse she would have trouble with typing and practical procedures such as bandaging or using scissors when her medication started to wear off. Claire was open and honest about the impact of constipation on her and those around her. This wasn't a minor issue or inconvenience. She explained how it was uncomfortable and painful, caused bleeding, affected intimacy and restricted her enjoyment of life. She found it embarrassing and discovered nobody really wanted to talk about it. She also described how it impacted absorption and efficacy of her medication. One symptom worsening other symptoms is a common experience in PD. Andrew described in poignant detail the distress he suffered from frequent dyskinesia, and how the uncontrollable, writhing-type movements of his whole body would leave him quite exhausted and influenced how others related with him. Ali conveyed how having a masked-like face meant that he could no longer show a natural smile. This always makes him very nervous when he meets patients for the first time as his facial expressions can be misinterpreted as depression or unfriendliness.

Nick addressed the symptom of fatigue. He articulated how difficult it is to adequately communicate this with others and convey that it is more than just a feeling of tiredness but an overwhelming lack of energy affecting the simplest of tasks.

Clare, spoke softly about the impact of postural hypotension, describing how she can frequently and unexpectedly feel dizzy as her blood pressure drops. She must be very careful and considered when changing posture such as standing up from a chair or getting out of a car to avoid feeling faint. Ed described his most bothersome Parkinson's symptom as muscle rigidity. He explained that his muscles were always switched on and never relaxed, causing aches and pains. His sometimes limped and his arm swing was reduced when he walked. Lorrie painted a picture of disrupted sleep. She recounted that it would start well but by two o'clock she was awake ticking off the hours. She described the immense relief at reaching six o'clock when she could at last get up. Finally, I attempted to describe what it felt like to wear off my medications and my frustration at how non-motor symptoms made me become hesitant and distant.

The film finished with the line, 'And that's why personalised care is key.' Ten different people with ten different symptoms. The collective effect of everyone's insight painted a picture of the challenge and complexity of living with PD. We entitled this film 'All the Same But Different.' Once more, we uploaded it onto YouTube and posted it on social media on 11 April 2022, World Parkinson's Day.

Advocacy is a common term in the Parkinson's community. It stems back to the Latin word *advocare* which means 'call to one's aid' and can be viewed as any activity which aims to make the lives of people better by bringing about sustained change.

Traditionally it is evidenced, in large scale and on a national level, in the form of Parkinson's charities that are continually striving for change. Much of the work goes unseen, but it is happening. Whether it is through funding for projects, provision of local support services, education or lobbying to scrap prescription charges and ensure all Parkinson's patients get their medication on time, they are advocating daily. But advocacy functions most efficiently in collaboration with those living with the condition. Each lived experience is unique, and whether that experience is positive or negative it engenders a voice, and we can determine to use it. Doing so does not diminish suffering or lessen impairment, but it does add meaning to our experience and ensures that our unique insights contribute to the bigger picture. When we empower our voice to bring about change for the better then we all become advocates, and our stories become resources. I was given a great piece of advice when diagnosed to endeavour, for as long as I am able, not to rely on others to advocate for me but to begin the process with myself. Even alone our voice has effect. I have witnessed that in the impact many individuals have had on different stages of my journey.

I first met Joy Milne when we were both guests on Larry's podcast in Kyoto. Joy is a retired nurse whose husband Les had Parkinson's. Demonstrating that scientific discoveries can be patient or carer led, she realised that she was able to identify an odour coming from him that no one else could smell. Joy has inherited a condition from her grandmother called hyperosmia, which means that she has a heightened sense of smell. When I heard the mesmerising story about how the scientific community designed a small experiment to prove if she could smell if someone had Parkinson's or not, I was intrigued. She was asked to smell the T-shirts of twelve different people in twelve different rooms. Six of the twelve had been diagnosed with Parkinson's previously and six had not. After Joy had completed the task, she said that seven of the twelve had Parkinson's and five did not. When that person was diagnosed eight months later it was proven that she got them all right. Since Les passed, she has dedicated her time and life work to advancing the understanding of PD, exploring new possibilities for diagnosis and moving beyond conventional thinking in the field of research. At seventy-four years she is an honorary lecturer in analytical olfaction at the Manchester Institute of Biotechnology at Manchester University and working hard. After Kyoto, I have kept in touch with Joy, and we have a WhatsApp video call a couple of times a year just to catch up. How she has taken her individual and unique insights and used them with determination to benefit others has been inspirational. Her story has become an amazing resource.

We don't have to change the world to change a life, and it can happen from a chair in our living room or coffee shop. However, if we can find ways of bringing together different voices then the capacity for change amplifies. The greater the number of pixels on a camera the clearer the image produced and so too is the strength of a co-operative.

As healthcare professionals living with Parkinson's these short films were made specifically to help educate our families, work colleagues and others in the NHS, but they had ignited a desire to use the unique perspective of the group in a way that would lead to effective change. The strength of our group is that we are not only living with Parkinson's but through all our various roles we have a good understanding of healthcare systems and how to bring about change within them, and I knew there was huge potential. However, I was aware of the scale of the challenge confronting us. To be a good advocate you need to face setbacks and keep persevering. It requires energy, motivation, resilience, determination, stubbornness and keeping your eyes on the goal – all things which can be challenging for those living with PD. Small differences may add to big change, but how often, for example, when we receive an email from a charity asking us to raise an issue with our MP do we respond? Overcoming inertia to start is often the hardest part.

Furthermore, it is not easy to make your voice heard in the realm of public health because of the sheer multitude of other voices with equal validity. Time and energy need to be focused at the right time, in the right manner and to the right place and people: towards those whose role is crucial to the outcome of how well someone with Parkinson's lives, such as care partners and employers and in the direction of those with vested interest, policy and decision makers in government and healthcare systems. I recognised that the secret would be to pick one topic, focus on it and persist until change happened. But with so many, which would be chosen?

CHAPTER 17

La Sagrada Familia

When the email arrived in my inbox in June 2022 it looked like any other from the WPC except for the words: 'Invitation to Participate' in the title. It certainly caught my interest, and I opened it with intrigue. Participate could have meant many different things from helping to run a workshop, getting involved in a roundtable discussion, to even facilitating a parallel session, but as I read the email in full it became clear exactly what the WPC had in mind. The Program Committee had invited me to give a plenary talk in the opening session of the 6th World Parkinson Congress (WPC 2023) due to be held in Barcelona, Spain, the following year.

My talk would be the last one of the four that morning. It is usual practice in these plenary sessions for the first three talks to be given by clinicians and researchers who are well respected in their field. The fourth one is usually earmarked for someone with Parkinson's to provide the perspective of lived experience. But when I first read the title 'What do subtypes mean for people with Parkinson's?' my heart sank. I had almost no knowledge about Parkinson's subtypes, never mind what they might mean for those living with the condition, and yet I needed to prepare a twenty-minute talk about them for an audience packed with clinicians, scientists and patients. I felt apprehensive at the enormity of the challenge.

Recognising that preparation was key I spent weeks searching the medical literature for journals, downloading them, reading them and underlining the key points. I was looking for themes to draw out and build up a picture of subtypes. However, it quickly became evident that the task would be difficult as there was no clear consensus about subtypes or their classification, and they remained poorly defined. Subtypes are a complex and developing facet of PD, a theoretical construct not yet established in clinical practice, and drawing context and relevance for those with PD would not be easy.

I wrote and rewrote my slides several times seeking to create a coherent link, but the talk just wouldn't come together. I was mindful of the need to balance the content as I would be speaking not only to Parkinson's healthcare workers and clinical researchers but also to people with Parkinson's and care advocates. I wanted to find a way to communicate detailed medical information to those who didn't understand medical jargon so that they would leave informed. However, much like explaining Parkinson's to my children, it is tough to simplify a complex subject without becoming simplistic.

DOI: 10.1201/9781003600671-17

I have attended many conferences over the years and was also aware that the audience's attention would be waning by the end of the session with three highly detailed medical talks, full of graphs and data, before mine. To be the last speaker is always a tough gig. I recognised the start of the talk would be key in determining the level engagement and that visuals would help sustain it.

After weeks of reflection the idea dawned to link the talk with the location, incorporating the essence of Barcelona as a city: something the audience would recognise and relate to and which I could somehow connect to subtypes. There was no shortage of options. Barcelona is a city associated with sport not just because of FC Barcelona and the skill of Lionel Messi but also for hosting the 1992 Summer Olympics. It is also a city with a deep architectural history evidenced even on a simple stroll through the streets. In 1999 it became the first city in the world to be awarded the Gold Medal for Architecture by the Royal Institute of British Architects.

Despite the wealth of possibilities by January 2023, the talk had no beginning or end and very little in between. As part of my research, I had been studying the history of architecture in Barcelona and couldn't get past the sheer beauty of one building that captivates, draws you in and lets your imagination run wild. It was La Sagrada Familia, the largest unfinished church in the world, designed by Antoni Gaudi.

'Why don't you use La Sagrada Familia as the basis of the talk?' Heather suggested one Thursday morning as we sat at our usual table with our familiar order of a large latte and a freshly made pot of Earl Grey tea. 'I don't think I could construct an entire twenty-minute talk on one building,' I replied. I had previously toyed with the idea but quickly rejected it. However, time was running out and a decision had to be made as I needed to submit a synopsis to the WPC the following week so I decided to explore the option further.

Although I had looked at lots of pictures of La Sagrada Familia, I had never been inside it. We had been in Barcelona for one morning and afternoon, many years ago, and had decided the quickest and most efficient way to see the main sites was to hop onto one of those red city sightseeing buses that grace the avenues of all major European cities. We had just enough time before our evening train to leave the bus and visit one site, but there was a dilemma. Heather wanted to explore the magic of La Sagrada Familia and I wanted to disembark at FC Barcelona's home ground, the Nou Camp. Both were full of history but for very different reasons. It wasn't a critical matter, so we decided to settle it fairly with the toss of a coin. 'Heads for the church, tails for the football,' I called as the coin flipped. Catching it firmly in my right hand and securing it onto my left I silently held my breath and hoped. It was tails. Delightedly I was heading to the Nou Camp. I really wanted to shout out 'Tails' as loudly as I could to celebrate, just like the Spanish football commentators shout 'GOALLLLLLLLLL' but I restrained myself and instead promised Heather that if we returned we wouldn't leave Barcelona without visiting La Sagrada Familia.

We had a second coffee order that morning, brainstorming ideas, and as we did so the beginning of possibility emerged. The more I read about Gaudi the clearer it became that if I incorporated comparisons between the building, Gaudi and Parkinson's, then this talk might just work. The key was taking these three threads, relating them to the subtypes and communicating them in a visual way that was simple to follow. I wanted to use the most iconic, pristine high-definition photos that I could find of the cathedral, both inside and out, to showcase what a showstopping building it was. It would be challenging but I knew they would look amazing projected on the huge auditorium screens. To aid my search I wrote directly to the Sagrada Foundation, explaining that I was presenting at the World Parkinson's Congress in Barcelona in July 2023 and that I wanted to base my talk on the cathedral. I didn't know if they would grant my request, but when the reply to my email dropped into my inbox I was taken aback. As I scanned the email, I couldn't quite believe what they were asking but on reflection it made sense. They were willing to grant permission for me to use their amazing photos but wanted the full text of my talk to ensure that it was in keeping with the values of the Sagrada Foundation. I typed my reply informing them that I would ensure they would be referenced throughout and that I would happily send the finished script. If they didn't agree that would be the end of the talk before it had even started.

I worked on the talk every Thursday. Never had I put so much effort into a single talk.

Eventually July arrived and we boarded the flight to Barcelona. We had decided to travel a few days earlier so we could have a short break and do some sightseeing. On the first morning we took the cable car up to the castle where we were able to survey the vista of the whole city. In the middle was the cathedral, rising in all its majesty. It really is the jewel in Barcelona's crown and we were both really excited at the prospect of visiting. We then walked to the Olympic stadium and took a moment to picture the 1992 100 m final. For the next two days we explored, shopped and visited various museums soaking up the art and culture. A highlight was the visit to La Padera (also known as Casa Mila), a residential property which Gaudi had designed. Beautiful on the outside, intricate in the inside, his creativity and capacity to incorporate nature in his designs, combining it with functionality, were a joy to behold. I particularly liked his door handles for left-handed people. It further heightened our anticipation to visit La Sagrada, which we had prebooked for our last morning in central Barcelona before we transferred to the convention centre. We had ensured this was organised before leaving Leicester as we didn't want to be disappointed.

As a couple Heather and I very much conform to the adage 'opposites attract.' I am an extrovert, she's an introvert, I do things straight away whereas she will procrastinate. . . . Inevitably there are occasions when such differences lead to conflict but equally the same differences can serve to balance each other's perspective.

Each of our eyes has a physiological blind spot. This is the part of the visual field where vision is not possible because of the absence of light-detecting photoreceptor cells in the region of the retina where the optic nerve passes through the optic disc. With both eyes open, the blind spots are not perceived because the missing information from one eye is filled in by the other. In life our 'subjective' perspective is like a single eye. There are things which we don't see or miss, not because they don't exist or aren't true, but because of a metaphorical 'blind spot.' We need another 'eye,' another 'objective' perspective, to provide the missing data that will complete the picture. Throughout our marriage Heather has acted as my 'other eye,' as I have for her, but this dimension of our relationship has certainly increased since I was diagnosed with PD. Non-motor symptoms seem, at times, to extend my blind spot. Dopamine is involved in multiple cognitive pathways in ways we do not fully understand, and there are impacts of this condition which are difficult to conceptualise and articulate. Over time I have developed self-awareness of a tendency to sometimes miss things in the bigger picture when I am focusing on the detail of a particular project. It is a tenuous symptom which comes and goes, but the most difficult aspect is that I don't recognise it. The inherent difficulty of an increasing blind spot, as the very name suggests, is that we can't see it. To counter this I regularly check with others and particularly Heather, to ensure I am not missing something obvious or that I have maintained correct vision of an issue or situation.

Living with PD is a humbling experience. We all like to believe we can function autonomously without help. No one relishes having to depend on others. But I have learnt that if I embrace the reality that I need help, then, far from limiting me, it will empower me. The alternative to not seeking help is to rely upon myself. But as my resources became restricted or diminished by the constraints of pathology, I have noticed the creep of anxiety that silently undermines confidence. Asking for help acts as a security net, liberating me to do more than I might otherwise.

And so, in the evening before we were due to relocate from central Barcelona to the convention centre, I ran through the full presentation. Although we had discussed it over several morning coffees, Heather had not heard it in completion, and I wanted to run it past her. It is difficult to describe what ensued in the following twenty-four hours, but it was a definite nadir of my experience with PD. When she listened to the presentation Heather suggested that whilst all the individual cogs were present, they were not aligned or coupled correctly. The result was that the presentation was disjointed and not flowing as smoothly or coherently as I had intended. She also voiced concern that my role as the fourth speaker was to bring together the topic for those at the conference with PD and she wasn't sure that I accomplished that.

It had been a very hot day in Barcelona, and I had probably overstretched myself in sightseeing. Our younger days of leaving the hotel early in the morning to spend hours exploring a city are no longer manageable, and we always ensure we return in the hotel in the early afternoon to rest for a least an hour before venturing out again in the evening. We had done that on this day but the heat and the walking from the previous two days had caught up and I was feeling especially symptomatic that afternoon. I was also extremely nervous about this presentation. I may have been used to speaking to full lecture theatres, but this was conference speaking on a big scale. Furthermore, the unique blend of speaking to professionals and patients at the same time and all of them experts in PD made it even more challenging.

The prospect of having to restructure and rewrite a presentation less than 48 hours beforehand tipped all my symptoms – both motor and non-motor – into overdrive, and the more symptomatic I became the more my ability to think and focus diminished and the more my anxiety spiralled. It was a perfect storm.

I knew I had to change slides, add new ones and update the script. My previous talk had been well rehearsed so I would also have to run through it a few times to make sure I didn't confuse the two. As my anxiety levels rocketed, I entered complete panic mode, pacing across the hotel room. I felt under so much pressure I thought my head would explode. I wasn't going to be familiar with this new talk. What if my mind couldn't process the words and I verbally froze standing in front of a large conference hall. I was worried how on earth we would complete it in time and there was no back-up. Heather quietly explained what needed to change and reassured me this would be easily fixed and that I had put too much work in to give up at this stage. So, in the bar of the hotel armed with tapas, we began the task of re-editing the talk.

I was so unwell that a process that should normally have taken a few hours seemed insurmountable. I didn't sleep and by 10 am the following morning, an hour before the taxi was due to take us to La Sagrada, the talk was still in disarray, my dopamine levels at rock bottom and my medications were having little impact. At 10.30 we looked at each other, resigned to the fact that we weren't going to make it to La Sagrada Familia for the second time. We rang to try and transfer the tickets to a later time but there was no space and there was no option but to cancel. The irony of spending months staring at photos to miss out on the real thing was a bitter pill for both of us to swallow. But PD was ruling the moment, and despite the best laid plans and intentions we left Barcelona for a second occasion without visiting the La Sagrada.

Within a few hours we had finalised the slides. It had taken so long that it was time to check out of our hotel room and move to the conference hotel. To overcome the fear of freezing we decided that using presenter view would be a good idea, but because the talk was new, I needed notes, and that meant I had to start transferring the script to the notes section of the presentation. So, we sat in the hotel foyer for a further three hours completing the task. When I pressed save for the final time, we jumped in a taxi and transferred to the conference hotel.

After checking into our room on the sixteenth floor, I looked out the window and over the city, rattled by what had happened. We attended the opening ceremony that evening as planned but when I was invited to gatherings afterwards, I politely declined. I was exhausted. I ran through the talk a few more times until it sounded as if it had been written months before and before nine o'clock was fast asleep.

The next morning, I woke up with an incredible sense of peace. I felt rested and ready. When the plenary session started, I listened intensely to the three talks before, which were packed with graphs and data. As the third speaker finished and walked back towards the table where all the speakers were sitting, I got up from my chair being careful not to trip. It felt like a long walk into the unknown which gave me time to ascertain that the audience needed a little interaction to refresh their concentration levels. It would take a few moments for my slides to be projected onto the screens, so I took the opportunity to ask them to wave at me. I wanted to take a photo for the kids to show them how many people I was talking to. They complied with smiles and laughter; I could feel the energy in the room lift and that in turn relaxed me. Although not the usual way to start a conference speech it was just what I needed. I glanced at Heather who, after the previous forty-eight hours, was now far more nervous than me, put my phone down and started to speak.

> Four years ago, I travelled to Japan and sat as a delegate in Kyoto to be inspired, encouraged and educated. I consider it a great privilege to be speaking to you this morning though to be honest it's a little daunting. When I heard that this congress was taking place in Barcelona, I was really looking forward to visiting. This city is full of two things I love, art and architecture, and perhaps the most iconic of all the architectural buildings must be La Sagrada Familia.
>
> It's a complex and intricate building. It has been shaped by the vision of one man, the genius architect, Antoni Gaudi. It has been worked on for a long time, by many master craftsman and each person's experience is individual and unique. As I was preparing this talk it struck me that it was very similar to Parkinson's. This is also complex and intricate. It was described from the observation of one man, James Parkinson. It has been studied for a long time by many master scientists and clinicians and everyone's personal experience is unique. I'm going to draw on these parallels throughout.

In full stride, all my anxiety dispelled, I continued. Even when a technological hitch meant a carefully considered video which was embedded at the end of the talk as the climax didn't play, I was able to calmly stop, wait for it to be fixed and finish as I had intended. To end, I thanked the audience for listening and acknowledged the Sagrada Foundation for approving the content of the talk in the weeks running up to the WPC. As the applause started, some people got to their feet, both those with Parkinson's and people from the scientific community, and I knew I had struck a chord with the audience. I looked at Heather and she smiled at me. She had spent hours patiently helping me craft and refine the talk and willingly sacrificed our trip to La Sagrada.

We live in a heavily filtered world, and it is difficult to be sure whether our judgements are accurate, as we can't always depend on the veracity of the information being presented to us. It is a danger of social media to overly focus on the positive and good, quietly airbrushing out the blemishes. When I suggested writing this book Heather had one immediate comment: 'You need to keep it honest.'

Whatever the external appearances there is always a cost of PD. It is possible to present a positive image so that everything looks good, but check carefully and you will discover that somewhere there is a filter. There are aspects of living with PD that are just hard and rubbish and that should be acknowledged. It is important in seeking to counter fatalism that the pendulum does not swing into toxic positivity. No matter how well we adapt, difficulties are always there, and it is disingenuous to deny them.

I know many people looked at me on that stage that morning and observed one version of PD. But a day earlier they would have witnessed a completely different one. Delivering the talk, I was riding the crest of a wave, but the day before I had been pummelled to the sea floor. We are only ever looking at one part of a whole.

It can be easy to misconstrue my high levels of activity and to envy what looks like productivity. I am on the go from 6 am, spending the day engaged in work and projects, accomplishing lots of tasks. But what is harder to perceive is the underlying drive of a brain chronically depleted and desperate to get more dopamine, and the reward or completion of a task provides just that. In one sense it's a craving, not for a drug, but for a neurochemical that will for a brief transient moment provide some relief. Ask me to sit and relax and to take pleasure in the moment and you will observe the issue more clearly. To enjoy a slow, lazy morning after a lie-in, reading the papers and eating brunch is no longer a choice – it is a fading memory of a life once lived. Heather is constantly seeking inventive ways to get me to sit in a garden chair and absorb some Vitamin D on a summer's afternoon. Two years ago, she discovered an app that identifies the birds in the garden. That succeeds in keeping me in a seat for twenty minutes whilst satisfying the dopamine hit of identifying new birdsong. But even then, it is never long before the restlessness and motor agitation that makes me want to move has me on my feet again or the urge to complete a task that has popped into my mind has me back at my computer or on my phone. For healthcare professionals this is difficult to assess – a clinic appointment is a twenty-minute snapshot – but succeed in identifying it and it will often point to areas where a patient or their care partner need help in the process of adaptation. A good question to always ask is, 'What is the cost of your PD in your daily life and for your relationships?'

A final point worth highlighting from this time in Barcelona is the reminder that unlike some conditions the impairment of PD is not fixed. If someone has a stroke or suffers an injury it can lead to a functional impact, but that tends to remain the same through the day and from one to the next. PD displays much greater fluidity and fluctuation. This makes planning hard because you can't always predict which version will present on a given day. But it also provides hope for the difficult days. That afternoon in the hotel my symptoms were as bad as they have ever been and yet two days later they were barely visible on a stage. This means that when I am facing a tough day I know the next is a new one and that it starts with a blank canvas. Some days the picture by dusk will be bleak and full of dark colours, some days the image will be sunny and vibrant, and some will have elements of both.

Chapter 18

Time Critical Medication

On a Saturday morning late in December, a bang of the front door signalled my opportunity. Mum had just left, probably on a festive errand, and Dad was nowhere to be seen. Within seconds and swift as a hare, I was on my hands and knees creeping covertly towards the pile of presents neatly stacked beneath the Christmas tree. Glancing at the labels to confirm I had located the correct pile and committing to memory the exact order and precise arrangement, I would inspect each present carefully, considering its shape, texture and noise when shaken. If the contents remained a mystery, I would prise apart the wrapping paper or create the smallest of tears at a corner before carefully replacing them all exactly as I had found them.

I have never been great at waiting, and the lessons of delayed gratification were hard learnt during childhood. I prefer tasks where I see results quickly. Give me a fence to paint or a border to dig but don't ask me to plant bulbs in the middle of autumn or sow seeds on a tray. And yet, like it or not, I have had to learn that the process of adaptation has far more in common with the latter. Learning, grieving and reframing core beliefs that have been established over years takes time. The process of adaptation is slow, incremental and often happens undetected. It requires an element of faith, trusting that the fruit of labours will happen at some point in the future even when there is little evidence of them in the present. Work must be done, and effort expended in expectation and when it is hard going, perseverance and endurance are essential to reach the goal, until one day realisation dawns that what was previously new has become established, what was atypical has become typical and what was exceptional has become mundane. The endpoint of adaptation is normalisation and is typically detected not at the time of occurrence but with reflective hindsight. One day you look back and suddenly realise the change has happened, that metamorphosis has taken place.

It was another winter morning and this time I was walking through majors on the way to a meeting when movement, behind the glass screen of one of the cubicles, caught my attention. I paused and observed that the patient within was visibly tremoring and gesturing to indicate she had something to tell me. I slid the screen, opening the cubicle, but her voice was weak and I had to approach the bedside to hear what she was saying. 'I have Parkinson's, and I need my medication,' she entreated in the quietest of voices, struggling to complete the sentence. I crouched down to ensure she could hear me. 'So do I and I am going to help you,' I whispered in response. She grabbed my right hand and gave it the tightest squeeze she could muster.

DOI: 10.1201/9781003600671-18

I left the cubicle and went to check her entry on the ED computer system and locate her notes. (At this point we had not yet transitioned to a paperless system.) A yellow 'Get It On Time' sticker had been placed on the front of her notes by the reception staff, to alert the nurses and doctors that she had Parkinson's and would need her medication administered at specific times while she was in the department. I could see she had last been prescribed a dose of levodopa at six o'clock the previous evening. However, there was no recorded evidence of her usual Parkinson's medication schedule in her notes, and when I checked her repeat prescriptions on the electronic system I could see that two morning doses had already been missed. None of her regular PD medications had been prescribed apart from the six o'clock dose of levodopa the evening before.

It is standard practice in the ED to only prescribe emergency medications such as antibiotics for sepsis, intravenous fluids, oral and intravenous pain relief and medication for cardiac arrhythmias. Patients are supposed to be processed through our department within four hours and once they are referred under the inpatient team, clinical responsibility is transferred to the admitting team, so it is not considered necessary to prescribe regular medications. However, Emergency Departments struggle daily with exit block. This is when all the beds in the hospital are filled and there is no capacity to move patients who are awaiting admission to the wards. The result is that the ED becomes overcrowded and a queue forms. It can often be many hours and sometimes days before they are finally transferred. Moreover, the ward teams are busy so it can take time for their doctors to come down into the ED to clerk in those waiting to be admitted and prescribe their regular medications. This frequently means that patients, as in this scenario, may miss their medications. Straightaway, I prescribed all her Parkinson's medication, not just the next dose.

This encounter bothered me. Presently, I am blessed to remain able to advocate for myself, but I understand the day will come when it could be me in that cubicle. With time an increasing eagerness to understand all perspectives of PD has taken root and galvanised a determination to identify ways in which care could be improved and endeavour to bring about change. I was therefore keen to establish how frequently doses were missed in our department and whether this patient's experience was unusual or representative.

The individuality of PD doesn't just apply to symptoms, it also applies to medication. Everyone has a unique and bespoke regime. Even if two patients are prescribed the same drug and dose, they may take them at different times, and the timing of doses in PD is critical. There are many medications whereby a missed or delayed dose will not cause any noticeable impact to either the patient or their condition because of the pharmacology of the drug. But there are other medications which are rapidly broken down and whose effects are immediate and important for function or survival. In these scenarios timing becomes an important factor. Ideally Parkinson's medication should be administered within thirty minutes of when it is prescribed. This is because once administered the levels of levodopa reduce quickly and as soon as they fall symptoms re-emerge.

A missed dose therefore prolongs the period of wearing off and increases the risk of complications such as falls. It can also contribute to an increased length of stay. By the time patients finally reach the wards stiffness and reduced mobility due to missed medication may necessitate physiotherapy input and delay discharge. Swallowing can become affected and voices weaken. If multiple doses are missed patients may need to be admitted to Intensive Care and may not survive. Lives are at stake and time really does matter – it's critical.

Parkinson's UK highlighted this important issue more than twenty years ago when it launched its 'Get It On Time Campaign' aiming to raise awareness within the healthcare system of the harm that is caused to individuals with PD when doses are delayed or missed. This had varying degrees of uptake across the UK. In 2019 the campaign was relaunched after a detailed report for England and Wales and one for Scotland indicated a systemic problem remained. Only forty-two percent of people with Parkinson's reported that they had received all their Parkinson's medication on time whenever they were in hospital, and, in 2018–19, it was estimated that there were 28,500 excess bed days in England and Wales, with one of the contributing factors cited being a delay in patients with PD receiving their medication. These reports did not get the in-reach that they deserved, as a few months later COVID was predominating headlines and the priorities in the NHS had immediately changed.

Although the NHS Professionals Living with Parkinson's Group was primarily set up for mutual support we often found ourselves discussing issues such as this as a group of professionals. We understand the impact of delayed medication on our own symptoms. We appreciate what a difference taking them even fifteen minutes later than planned can make: how a missed dose can ruin a family day out, how symptoms worsen but don't necessarily recalibrate with the next dose, sometimes persisting for one to two days. We couldn't begin to imagine what it was like for those in hospital, in a vulnerable position and already unwell, not to receive their medications when needed, but we could imagine their anxiety and fear. A hospital should be an environment that facilitates healing, recovery and rehabilitation, not one that harms or causes a decline from baseline and certainly not because of something as simple as patients not receiving their medication when they usually take it.

We wanted to help but understood that although the problem appeared simple it was far more complex: hence the reason it remained a problem twenty years after first being highlighted. We knew we could add value to the debate, that between us we had years of training and experience in healthcare and that we held a unique position to understand the complexity from both sides of the coin. The bigger question was how to help and in such a complex matter where to start. Clare A suggested that we should establish a working group and eleven of us decided to meet virtually. As we began to observe our various places of work it was clear the same issues were emerging time and again. Patients who were asleep were not being woken, medications were not being administered according to the prescribed times because nursing staff were busy with other issues and individuals were experiencing unnecessary symptoms as a result. We decided to embark on a campaign with three distinct phases.

Our primary aim was to translate words into action. We did not want to simply replicate the good work already being done. We wanted to advocate for patients in hospitals across all four nations to receive their Parkinson's medications within thirty minutes of when they needed them in a manner that converted ideals into measured improvements in outcome. This was a huge undertaking. What we were seeking to do was to challenge convention and change culture, not just in one hospital or one region or one nation but across the NHS in England, Scotland, Wales and Northern Ireland. It would depend upon engaging the right people in the right places across various aspects of the healthcare and charitable sectors.

Our first objective was to clarify messaging. Our research had indicated that even if staff grasped the general need for medications to be administered on time they were not aware how short the window of delay was before potential harm could arise and that administrations even thirty minutes later than the person with Parkinson's would normally take them could prove impactful. We decided it was essential to emphasise the importance of this time factor. We have all worked in busy departments and comprehend the enormous demands on staff from so many directions – demands which far outweigh both their time and their resources. There are multiple standards and ideals to be upheld, and staff must constantly prioritise and discern what is most urgent and where the need is greatest. We understood that to break through the clamour of voices calling for improvements our message would need to be simple, be clear and communicate urgency.

The group decided to complement the long-running Parkinson's UK 'Get It On Time' slogan by creating an angle that pressed home the exigency of this issue in healthcare settings, using the simple term Time Critical Medication (TCM). We hoped that highlighting this would begin to shift the perception from an ideal to a clinical need, knowing that all NHS professionals will more readily engage when they understand that patient well-being underpins what they are being asked to change. We also identified that previous reports had only considered ward settings. However, we were keen to broaden the scope of the issue, highlighting that TCM needs to be on everyone's agenda – admin staff, doctors, nurses and pharmacists – from the minute the patient accesses the NHS to when they are discharged.

Phase One of the campaign was launched on World Parkinson's Day, 11 April 2022, with the release of a short three-minute video on social media called 'Time Matters: It's Critical.' Its purpose was to educate and introduce the concept of TCM.

We created an ideal patient journey from arrival to an ED. This included being identified at the outset as a patient taking TCM, establishing quickly what medication is usually taken, ensuring that all Parkinson's medication is prescribed, not just their next dose, and finally administrating the doses within thirty minutes. It was introduced by two NHS CEOs who acknowledged that when people with Parkinson's didn't get their medications on time it caused harm. A letter was then composed for every chief executive officer (CEO) of an acute hospital in England and every CEO of the health regions and boards in Scotland, Wales and Northern Ireland. The chief nursing officers of all four nations were also included as well as the NHS medical director for England and the chair of the Association of Ambulance Chief Executives. They would simply be asked to pledge their support to this campaign via email.

This sounded good in theory, but I was used to managing busy inboxes. How would we ensure that this letter that was to be emailed would stand out amongst the hundreds they received every week? I phoned every personal assistant to every CEO and explained what we were trying to achieve. They were all very happy to support us and give us their direct contact details. We then split up the hospitals amongst the group.

I also knew from experience that collaborative working will always be more likely to advance an issue and was keen to create consensus and ensure joined-up thinking between our NHS professional group and Parkinson's UK.

At this point in time, the Parkinson's Excellence Network (a group of health and social care professionals, supported by Parkinson's UK, working to share best practice to educate and drive improvements in services for those with PD) was running four national priority programmes, based on feedback from their two-year national audit. One of these priorities was to revisit 'Get It On Time' and build on the work that had already been started through the first campaign and 2019 report. Clare and I were invited to join this working group representing the work of the NHS Professionals group and to promote co-operation. When the pledges were returned to our group via email from CEOs, they were followed up by the Parkinson's UK local campaign officers in England and the service improvement managers in Scotland, Wales and Northern Ireland. There was debate over whether the slogan 'Get It On Time' should be replaced by 'Time Critical Medication,' but following discussions it was agreed that when dealing with NHS professionals the programme would be referred to as TCM, but when dealing with the general public the slogan Get It On Time would continue to be used.

By the end of the first year of the campaign, we had received over one hundred pledges of support from CEOs of acute healthcare trusts and regional ambulance services, the chief nursing officers and other NHS executives across all four nations, including the national medical director of NHS England. We understood that it was only the beginning and would take years to see measured improvements, but it was encouraging to know that Time Critical Medication as an issue had crossed the desks of a lot of influential people within the healthcare system.

During the campaign I applied for a role within the Parkinson's Excellence Network and was delighted to be part of the Clinical Leadership Team. In collaboration with PEN and as part of my new role, Phase Two of our campaign was to write a document for NHS trusts, outlining ten recommendations that would support healthcare professionals in implementing Time Critical Medication management. This document formed part of a report produced by Parkinson's UK in September 2023 called 'Every Minute Counts: Time Critical Parkinson's medication on time, every time.' Key points raised included education of all staff to recognise that Parkinson's medication was time critical, the role of electronic prescribing to aid accurate and timely prescribing and the need to review the issue of self-administered medications. Again, we wrote to every CEO that we had written to the year before asking them to benchmark their acute NHS trust against the ten recommendations document. This work remains ongoing and we are continuing to actively engage with trusts.

Phase Three of the campaign was to get stakeholder engagement from the Medical Royal Colleges from within the NHS in the four nations of the UK and at government level.

In March 2023, Clare suggested that we should apply for a Health Service Journal (HSJ) Patient Safety award to help raise the profile of our objective. At first I was reluctant, as we weren't yet in the position of evidencing improvement in the numbers of patients receiving their Time Critical Medication within thirty minutes, but with reflection, I recognised there was nothing to lose. The application form was detailed but we managed to pull it together before the closing date, and when I received a WhatsApp message a few weeks later confirming we had been shortlisted, everyone was excited. This was an excellent opportunity for Time Critical Medication to be raised on a national level.

The next step was a vigorous twenty-five-minute face-to-face interview over Zoom with two HSJ award judges in which we had to present three reasons why we should win. I presented the first reason, which was that this entry was from a group of NHS professionals advocating for patients in hospital who also live with the same condition. Clare explained the second reason, which was that this project had three ambitious phases. Although Phase One had just been completed we were keen to show the judges the long-term strategy to improve and sustain safer care. Jean Almond, the programme manager of the PEN workstream on TCM, stated the third reason, which was that the award would be recognition for a group of NHS professionals who had volunteered their time to improve patient safety. Once the judges finished asking their questions, it was then a matter of waiting until the awards evening in September.

The day of the awards ceremony finally arrived and with a mixture of nerves and excitement I boarded an early train to Derby to speak in the morning at a conference about living with Parkinson's. There are two great things about speaking at such events. The first is meeting with other patients and sharing stories: every conference

I attend as a speaker I always leave having learnt something myself. The second is the opportunity it provides to connect with other healthcare professionals. I sit on the Parkinson's Excellence Network Clinical Leadership team with Fiona (Lindop), a physiotherapist, who had organised the conference. Over the years she has been a great encouragement, but working on national level projects means that meetings sometimes are offline, so it's always great to meet in person. After a quick lunch, it was back to the station for the onward train to Manchester and the award ceremony.

Overall, there were five hundred and six entries, with two hundred and six organisations and projects making it to the final shortlist, following two rounds of rigorous judging. We were proud to have reached this stage and were determined to enjoy the evening no matter what the outcome was. Clare had put in so much hard work and because it was such a big occasion she decided to fly back from her holiday in Greece to attend the awards ceremony, returning the next day. As I took my seat on the train, she messaged to say that she was just boarding her flight and would arrive about an hour beforehand. It was going to be a challenge for both of us to sustain dopamine levels throughout this day.

When I arrived in Manchester and checked in to my hotel, I rested and then caught up on some work emails, mainly to try and divert the growing mass of butterflies in my stomach. Eventually it was time to get changed. This was less straightforward than it sounds. Heather was not with me and the exercise of putting on both cufflinks and sorting my bow tie required trial, patience and perseverance, but I managed it.

Our entry was a collaborative one, Jean (the Time Critical Medication programme manager) and Grace (Campaigns Engagement lead) were representing PEN. Clare and Tincy, both nurses, would represent the NHS Professionals Living with Parkinson's Group. As I was formally working with the Parkinson's Excellence Network and a member of the group, there would be equal representation around the table. The HSJ awards venue was a stone's throw away from the hotel, and we had all agreed to meet in the foyer fifteen minutes before they started. 'Has everyone got their medications?' I gestured to Clare and Tincy, knowing it was going to be a long night, and checked mine for the third time.

There were twenty-four different categories and ours was scheduled to be the fourteenth one to be announced. The first part of the evening passed in nervous anticipation; I could almost feel the needle on the internal dopamine tank hasten towards zero, but we finally reached our category, the 'Patient Involvement in Safety Award.' We had agreed that if we won then Clare would accept the award as she had proposed the idea all those months ago. Seven entries had been shortlisted which to my calculations meant we had a fourteen percent chance of winning.

As the presenter walked to the podium I held my breath. Could a group of people living with a progressive, degenerative, neurological disease win a prestigious national award? Under the table, my left leg was doing a merry dyskinetic dance all on its own. He began:

> Good evening, everyone. The judges recognised the winning project's significance in enhancing patient involvement with positive feedback on engagement efforts and felt their presentation effectively highlighted stakeholder engagement, applauding how the campaign's clear three-phase approach included a range of issues, well done. And the winner is – The NHS Professionals Living and Working with Parkinson's.

Tincy let out the loudest 'Whoop' beside me that made me jump. Clare rapidly tapped her feet into the ground, Jean punched the air and Grace had the biggest smile on her face that ran from cheek to cheek. I couldn't quite believe it, I had doubted that it could be done, but I was proved wrong.

We all stood up and hugged each other, but very quickly the realisation dawned that we would have to walk to the stage. There were twenty-five tables of ten people and we were in the second row from the back. When three people with Parkinson's have to reach the front of the stage and climb up steps, it is going to take a bit longer than for your average person. As we started walking towards the stage the effects of the day had taken their toll and I was acutely aware of my symptoms. My left leg had become a dead weight and I felt as if a cannonball was chained to my ankle. The distance suddenly seemed to double and the closer we came the more I was worried about getting up the stairs without tripping. I did not relish the idea of falling in front of a room full of people whose eyes at that instant were all focused on the stage. In the end I managed but I was so symptomatic on stage that Jean linked arms to steady me. At that point I was very grateful for a helpful and understanding hand, and it assuaged enough of the growing anxiety to enable me to enjoy the moment. As Clare accepted the award, we posed for the official HSJ photographer to take our pictures and then we exited the stage to the left. We walked to applause along the side of the room feeling triumphant on one hand and hoping we would make it to the back without tripping on the other. We walked through a door at the back of the awards hall that took us to an interview area. It felt akin to being on the red carpet of the Oscars, with a backdrop of logos, a photographer snapping away and a film crew with their lighting shining brightly. 'Congratulations, so well deserved, how do you feel?' the interviewer asked. 'It feels really exciting,' Clare said looking around at us all. 'It is helping push this campaign to another level and that's fantastic,' she added.

This national endorsement by the HSJ highlighted the importance of Time Critical Medication as a patient safety issue and the role that all staff could play in ensuring that people with Parkinson's get their medications on time, every time, in hospital.

It was around eleven o'clock by the time the last award was finished and an announcement informed us that the room was about to be cleared in preparation to dance the night away. Without saying anything Clare, Tincy and I looked at each other and we knew that was the end of our night. There was little left in the tank for walking and none for dancing, and we were mindful that tomorrow would already be enough of a challenge.

The next morning as I headed back on the train to Leicester, I reflected how far I had travelled metaphorically. Eight years after diagnosis I had undertaken a hectic forty-eight-hour schedule that would have been challenging even for someone without PD, with taking four train journeys, speaking at a conference and attending a late-night awards ceremony. Putting on cufflinks had taken a while; I had needed to go longer between doses to sustain me until late into the evening, meaning an hour nap in the late afternoon was necessary. It had been a struggle to make it onto the stage and I had to skip the dancing, but the point was I had managed it and the adjustments I had made to do so had almost become reflex and instinctive. Life was not normal compared to ten years earlier, but it had normalised. If PD was the result of a single pathological incident, then this would have represented the end of the journey. But of course, stability in PD is illusionary. Parallel to the process of adaptation is that of degeneration. PD is dynamic, and it is impossible for anyone to reach the end of the process. Adaptation is lifelong. But what is possible is to experience periods where PD retreats from the foreground. Returning from Manchester I was filled with gratitude to find myself at one of those junctures.

Over the course of 2023–24 Phase Three of the campaign gained further momentum. Six months after the HSJ awards a Time Critical Medication proposal I had submitted to the Royal College of Emergency Medicine's (RCEM) Quality Improvement Programme (QIP) competition won. This three-year project would involve over one hundred EDs across the UK's four nations. As I had begun exploring the issue of Time Critical Medications, I had discovered that there was a broader scope than PD. Although the number is small, there are other medications where delayed or missed doses have significant impact. I recognised that the same processes we were attempting to implement would hold true for them and that if I extended the scope of this ED project to include other conditions, we would have more data points and gain more traction. There are only two conditions that require medications to be given within thirty minutes. One is Parkinson's and the other is insulin-treated diabetes. EDs were asked to submit three cases of each condition weekly. We had three standards which, if addressed, would lead directly to ensure that TCM would be given when the patient usually took them. We wanted to improve the time it took to identify that a person who attended an Emergency Department was on a Time Critical Medication. Once identified we wanted to ensure that all their medication was prescribed and administered in the ED, even if they were under the care of another inpatient team. Finally, we wanted patients with capacity to have the option of self-administering their medication.

In September 2023, Parkinson's UK officially launched the 'Every Minute Counts' report in Parliament, and they invited Clare and me to join them. It was an excellent opportunity to not only discuss with MPs the importance of Time Critical Medication for people with Parkinson's in hospital, it was also an opportunity to bring our oldest children with us to see advocacy in action.

Finally in May 2024 when the national medical director of NHS England announced a three-year Medicines Safety Improvement Programme (MEDSIP) for TCMs in hospital, we knew that the issue had reached the national agenda. We hope that NHS Scotland, Wales and Northern Ireland will all follow suit.

We know the key to improving the quality of care lies in three key things. Firstly, the addition of an electronic tagging system to quickly identify those on TCMs when they first arrive at the hospital. (An ED-specific TCM sticker for the front of the ED notes could be used in the meantime for paper-based departments until they switch over.) Secondly, by using electronic prescribing systems to record the administration of all Parkinson's medication, there would be an easily accessed and accurate database which could be analysed to identify where the delays were. Finally, we knew that if we got the first dose right in the ED, then the chances were that subsequent doses would be more likely to be given when the person with Parkinson's needed them.

There has been good progress in three years but there remains much work to do; however, we will endeavour to keep going because Time Matters: It's Critical. Changing the NHS is in many ways a form of adaptation and many of the same principles hold true. The process is slow, at times it can feel like nothing is happening and that you are labouring in vain, but it is important to hold faith and keep persevering in expectation that one day the seed will sprout and start to send up shoots, eventually producing fruit.

Welcoming in 2024 I felt in a better place than I had at any New Year since 2016. This was the year I turned fifty. My medication schedule had remained largely stable for twenty-five months, my side effects were well controlled and manageable, and I had found a routine in work and home that was enabling me to enjoy a better quality of function at fifty years than I had dared hope when I was diagnosed at forty-one years. But an important lesson from the period after I was first diagnosed had receded to the back of my mind – that PD is only one piece of the picture. There is a bigger perspective, and this was soon to forcefully reassert itself right back in the foreground of my thinking with the words, 'I'm sorry but you have cancer.'

CHAPTER 19

Co-Morbidities

Travelling through the blackness of a tunnel, there is less concept of speed than when the train emerges and the scenery whizzes past. The passage of time is judged by observing the landscape.

A few months ago, I was reminiscing with Ben about the impact of a favourite movie from my teens, *Dead Poets Society*. The discussion prompted me to purchase it and with some persuasion he reluctantly agreed to watch what I promised was a classic. However, time passes faster than we sometimes acknowledge and it's often only when we revisit a bygone era that we realise how much. Films can act as time machines suddenly flipping our perspective. So much had altered personally and in society from when I watched it in 1990 that the film did not have the same impact and Ben's viewpoint, as an eighteen-year-old, was different again. Perspective, as any artist or photographer will assert, is key.

With reflection my experience of adapting to illness started young, at the age of seven, when I was hospitalised several times with severe asthma. This led to skin testing that revealed an allergy to dust mite, pets and even my own hair. Radical changes to my bedroom followed. The mattress had to be sprayed with special medicine and placed in a protective cover twenty-four hours a day, seven days a week. The carpet was replaced with lino and the curtains with a blind: even the lightshade was removed and I had to keep my window open for a few hours every day. When I took my slippers off in the evening to get into bed, the floor was freezing. Sometimes it felt more like prison than a bedroom. I couldn't have that dog that I always wanted, though we did have plenty of goldfish. Goldfish, however, don't go for walks, chase a ball or interact with you. From an early age my perspective of life was informed by illness.

As a teenager and young adult, I began to grasp the need to adapt not only to manage present conditions but also potential future ones. From the moment we are conceived our health and function is influenced by our genetics. We can inherit mutations or combinations of genes which either directly cause or predispose us to illness. For the most part we have no idea what is written into the code of our DNA but occasionally there are glimpses of light that act as a beacon to redirect and steer us towards safer water.

My grandmother stood at the bus stop on a cold, foggy morning and blew a kiss. Little did she know it would be the last time she would see him alive. It was the 13th of

 DOI: 10.1201/9781003600671-19

February 1965, and my grandfather had just boarded the bus with other members of Banbridge rugby club to travel to Dublin to watch Ireland in the Five Nations rugby tournament at Lansdowne Road versus England.

As the bus pulled away, she put her hand inside her coat pocket pretending to pull something out and wave it at him. He realised that her gesture was to get him to check that he had the tickets. He put his hand into his coat pocket and waved them back at her. It was a low scoring game with Ireland scoring the only try to win 5–0. In high spirits after a famous win, everyone returned to the bus to travel home. Today the road connecting Banbridge to Dublin is a mix of motorway and dual carriage way, bypassing the large towns of Drogheda and Dundalk, and can be completed with ease in an hour. But back then it was a different matter. The main A1 meandered its way through towns and villages and the outer suburbs of Dublin and on an international match day when the volume of traffic moving across Ireland to Dublin was high, the journey could take three to four hours.

About halfway through the journey home my grandfather started to feel nauseated, developing central chest pain and sweating profusely. The pain intensified as the bus crossed over the border from the Republic of Ireland back into Northern Ireland and it was clear at the age of fifty-seven years he was having a massive coronary. An arteriosclerotic plaque within one of the arteries that supplied his heart had ruptured, causing a clot to form. As it increased in size less blood was reaching his heart muscle, starving it of vital oxygen. The bus diverted to the closest hospital but by the time he was helped inside it was too late; the doctors said there was nothing they could do. Back then, in the mid-1960s, there was no treatment to dissolve the clot in a blocked artery or open it up with a stent or a balloon to restore the blood flow and prevent the muscles from dying. He died just after midnight, on the 14th of February. My grandmother would never again receive flowers from him on that day, and instead the occasion of Valentine's Day would be marked when she placed flowers on his grave.

Close to a quarter of all deaths in Northern Ireland are due to heart and circulatory disease. This is in stark contrast to the Tsimané people of the Bolivian Amazon who, with a combination of a healthy diet and six hours of exercise a day, are thought to have the healthiest hearts in the world. But even accounting for geography, examination of our family history suggests a predisposition to ischaemic heart disease in our family genes. My grandfather had six brothers, four of whom died of heart disease in their fifties. My own dad had a stent inserted in two of his coronary arteries and his brother had a triple coronary artery bypass graft; Dad was in his early sixties, his brother in his fifties. I can't alter or fix my genetic make-up, but with education, monitoring and treatment of cardiovascular risk factors I can adapt my lifestyle to reduce the likelihood. I can choose to not smoke, modify what I eat, annually check my cholesterol, monitor my blood pressure and exercise regularly, and so I have been mindful of these things from an early age.

But even with the healthiest of lifestyle and the best of surveillance when it comes to the domain of health, nothing is certain. Some will manage significant ill health throughout their life, others very little. One illness does not preclude the possibility of others, and as I was soon to learn we don't have a quota for health.

In April 2024, I was showering, as I do, every morning. I am more of a top-down washer starting with my chest and abdomen, followed closely by my armpits with a final sweep of my bits down below. As I did this, I was acutely aware that my right testicle felt like a dead weight when compared to the left. When I examined it further it was clearly more than twice the size of the left one and felt hard, like a rock.

About four weeks earlier I had briefly questioned whether my right testicle was slightly larger than the left, but I recalled from learning anatomy in medical school that the right one could be slightly larger than the left, so I had dismissed it when I didn't notice it again the next day. (The reason I don't think I noticed the increase in size in the intervening four weeks was because I had begun regularly cycling in the morning as part of a group exercise challenge, prior to having my shower, and after exercise the skin around the testes can contract, lifting them upwards, and making them more difficult to feel when washing.) But this time my clinical instinct was on full alert and my head was spinning. I turned off the shower and explained to Heather that I needed to make an appointment with the GP.

To request an emergency appointment in our surgery requires phoning at 08.30 on the day the appointments are released. By now it was gone nine o'clock and when I registered that I was number forty-five in the queue I gave up any chance of obtaining an appointment that day and hung up deciding to retry in the morning, but I couldn't settle. Every cog in my brain was whirring. I tried to recall whether I might have injured it but couldn't think of anything. I located my pen torch to see if it shone in the dark, but it didn't. I got Heather to check but her quiet lack of reassurance told me all I needed to know – her own clinical instinct was now also on high alert. Nothing eased the growing sense of anxiety and of course the more anxious and stressed I became the more my non-motor symptoms began to emerge. I was distracted, restless, agitated and unable to quell the growing compulsion to get an answer as soon as possible. By eleven o'clock, Heather ascertained I was going to struggle to wait until the morning and suggested I phone on the off chance the surgery would have a late cancellation. I was so relieved when I finally cleared the queue to hear the receptionist inform me that there was indeed an appointment with an advanced practitioner at 2 pm. 'I will take that,' I replied without hesitation. When she asked about the problem I explained I had a swollen testicle. (No amount of medical training makes it feel any less strange or embarrassing talking about your anatomy over the phone.)

Any sense of relief I felt at getting an appointment was short lived when she quickly phoned me back to say that I needed to be seen by a GP. 'But don't worry,' she continued. 'We have made you an appointment to see one at 16.45 and he used to work as a urologist.' I couldn't quite believe it. It is unusual to encounter a urologist in a GP practice, but it was such a godsend to know I was effectively going to get a specialist opinion straight away. As I sat nervously in the waiting room, having read the leaflets pinned to the notice board for the third time, I knew what to expect from the consultation. During training I was taught, as all doctors are, how to examine a testicular swelling. First you see if you can get above the swelling. If you can't that means that a portion of bowel may have herniated into the scrotum through a breach in the muscle wall of the abdomen. That wasn't me. Next you see if the swelling is separate from the testicle by gentle rolling it between your finger and thumb. If it is, the most likely cause is inflammation of tissue that sits on top of the testicle. That wasn't me either. Finally, you turn out the lights and place a pen torch under the scrotum to see if fluid has accumulated in the scrotal sac. If it has then it lights up like a beacon. That wasn't me either. I had already examined and re-examined myself several times and I knew the swelling was coming from within the testicle. After the GP completed his examination, he explained that he would refer me for an urgent ultrasound scan and make an appointment with a urologist.

Ten days later, and eight years after I had been given my Parkinson's diagnosis, I walked once again along the corridor at the Leicester General Hospital. This time it felt longer than ever. I stopped to check my appointment location and followed the arrow, this time to urology, not neurology. When the urologist beckoned me into the room, I walked across the clinic floor with my arms swinging symmetrically and sat down on the chair bedside his desk having not scuffed my foot. He asked some questions and then he examined me. When he had finished, he looked up and nodded. He didn't have much to say. This time there was no seismic shock – Heather and I both knew it was testicular cancer, the most common male cancer in men aged between fifteen and forty-nine. I had snuck in there by six months as I would celebrate my fiftieth birthday in November.

As we drove home, we passed the kids' old primary school. They were both now at secondary school and growing up fast. Ben was sitting his A-levels in four weeks. We passed the church and my thought this time was whether I would even be alive on Anna's wedding day. We passed the golf course and all I could visualise was that my right testicle was the size of a golf ball. The following week I had a CT scan of my chest, abdomen and pelvis to determine if there was any spread but I wouldn't know exactly what I was dealing with until after my surgery.

This diagnosis was different to PD and in a way more straightforward. With testicular cancer I was in full blown attack mode. I wanted it removed as soon as possible. It felt like an invader and an unwelcome presence in my body. I hadn't been able to adopt the same principles when dealing with PD as it can't be removed and it can't be cured. It is difficult to frame PD as an enemy because it becomes part of who you are and I needed to find ways to manage it and live well with it. I remember the precise date and time I was diagnosed with PD, but the time and date I was diagnosed with testicular cancer is not engrained in my brain. The time and date of the surgery, however, is. On 29 April at 09.40 I was wheeled into theatre and when I woke up and

I was given my PD medication on time, when I would have usually taken them: two victories in one morning.

My post-operative recovery was a challenge. I developed a wound infection that delayed healing and required a course of antibiotics. But the bigger hurdle was the prolonged break from exercise to allow my wound to knit. 'Don't stress your wound. You don't want to give yourself a hernia,' had been my surgeon's parting words. Every aspect of the doctor within me understood that I had to give my body time to rest and recover. I have heard myself issue similar instructions so many times, but it is easier to preach than practice. It was difficult to suddenly transition from cycling fifty kilometres a week to none. Exercise is fundamental in the control of my PD symptoms, especially the non-motor ones, and so it was no surprise that cessation of all exercise eventually began to impact my function. When I closed my eyes all I could picture was my neurons sitting labile. Furthermore, I missed the endorphins, and I do not relish prolonged periods of rest. It makes me feel restless and agitated. In addition to discontinuing exercise, normal mobilisation had also become a struggle. I was surprised at the degree of pain I was experiencing, and the limitation in movement did little to help my motor symptoms increasing my stiffness.

Three weeks later the oncologist confirmed that I had Stage 2 testicular cancer and advised a cycle of chemotherapy. I was very apprehensive about how it would affect my symptoms. I especially feared sickness and vomiting knowing this would alter the absorption of my medication and could potentially be enormously detrimental. This is a quandary regularly facing patients and clinicians, the need to find a balance between two opposing tensions, the management needs of one condition versus the negative impact on the management of another. However sometimes balance is impossible, and possible deterioration must be accepted as a necessity. And this was the situation I found myself in. The long-term risk of not managing testicular cancer was a reduction in survival. The impact on my PD was reduction in function and quality of life. I may not like the latter, but it was simply no contest. For this moment in time PD had fallen down the agenda. To maximise the chance of achieving remission I had to accept it. This is the effect of perspective and how the big picture changes things. It is also why everyone's management of PD looks different. Not only is there variation in the presentation of the condition itself, there is enormous diversity in the big picture. What is possible for one person is not always achievable for the next. The ability to adapt depends on so many variables and what I learnt from my experience of testicular cancer is that whilst community and support circles and psychology all have an important influence, co-morbidities are arguably the biggest.

As I sat waiting to enter the chemotherapy suite to continue my treatment the irony of my position was not lost. How had I managed to get diagnosed with one condition at forty-one years of age which was more common in older people and one condition at forty-nine which was more common in younger people? It was a stark reminder that life doesn't follow textbooks.

Once called, I nervously entered the chemotherapy suite to a hive of activity. There was a row of recliner chairs lined up, one after another. There were people of different ages and different stages. Some had lost their hair, others hadn't. Some were there for the first time, others had been on this well-walked path for a while. I was greeted by one of the nurses who asked if this was my first time in the chemotherapy suite. It was obviously clear to people that it was. I had not brought anything to do. Someone was knitting, several were reading, others had brought their iPads, one was watching an episode of the sitcom *Friends*. The nurse inserted a cannula into the back of my hand and showed me to my recliner. As the drip containing the medication was attached, it slowing started to enter my body. I closed my eyes and said a prayer before sitting for an hour watching every drip.

Once the infusion had finished and the cannula was removed the oncology nurse gave me a prescription for some metoclopramide, an anti-sickness medication. 'I can't take that, as it interferes with my Parkinson's medication,' I said. 'What do you usually take instead?' she inquired. Once again, I was reminded of the need for further education for both healthcare professionals and those living with Parkinson's. I was able to advocate for myself because of education and the knowledge I had of important drug interactions with PD medications. I remembered back to the day I had started oral levodopa when my neurologist had prescribed three days of domperidone, which worked well. Thirty minutes later I was given a five-day supply and I left the suite hoping I would not need to return.

I was greeted by Heather and Ben, who had now finished his A-level exams. There were no words; we didn't have to say anything but just hugged. I took the anti-sickness medication every eight hours. They worked well and although I felt nauseated first thing in the morning, they helped to keep it at bay for the rest of the day.

I think what I missed most in the following weeks was my routine. For eight years I had been going to the gym early but I was too tired, and because I wasn't working I had lost the routine of going beforehand. It took four months in total to return to work. I had a repeat CT chest, abdomen and pelvis that still didn't show any evidence of spread and entered a five-year surveillance program with a chest x-ray and blood tests every six months alternating with a CT scan and bloods six months after that. Although I can usually put it out of my head, when these investigations come around again the thought of it coming back is never too far away.

It is not easy to adapt to a condition when you know that despite your best efforts there will be ongoing degeneration. When I turned forty and considered the span of the decade ahead, I was planning career progression, home improvements, a road trip to California and ways to improve my fitness. But when I learnt I had PD it was as though someone implanted a lens which coloured everything in my field of vision. In the absence of a cure or medications which modify the disease, the future suddenly looked bleak, and at first efforts to adapt felt futile. Was there really any point in getting up at 6 am every morning to go to the gym or eating healthily? It didn't prevent me getting PD and wasn't going to fix the problem now that I had it.

Honesty compels me to acknowledge that there are times when PD can feel like a disease that rains on our hopes and dreams, darkening the horizon with storm clouds. But just as a rainbow can appear in an unexpected arc, so too amongst the losses there are gains which add colour and bring beauty. And for me the two great gifts of PD have been the reframing of time and perspective. It is very easy in the business of life to pass and write things into our future in the expectation we will have one. We make plans to travel or take up a hobby when we have retired or visit that friend next month only to discover that the business crowds out next month's schedule also. But when the future is clouded, then the present takes on new value, and today becomes the imperative. And this helps us to take stock and realign priorities to determine what is important and to take enjoyment in the gift that is, today.

But as I adapted to PD and discovered a new normal, the tendency to revert to old patterns had returned. The storm clouds seemed less, the sky brightened and my perspective inevitably drifted once more. However, cancer restored my outlook and reminded me again of the value of time; the one commodity that is perpetually declining and which we can never reclaim. So, I make time to ensure coffee with Heather continues every Thursday. When the sun is shining, I sit in the garden to listen to the birdsong and I swing a golf club as often as possible because it brings me pleasure. I work hard because I am able and when the opportunity presented during a visit to Wales to divert an hour off a planned route to complete a zip line with Heather, Ben and Anna, I grasped the opportunity in front of me because when I looked carefully at that lens implanted in my vision after diagnosis, imprinted right across the centre was a phrase from *Dead Poets Society*. The movie may have dated but its famous quote has not – '*carpe diem*' – seize today.

CHAPTER 20

Enabling Not Disabling

Historically Parkinson's disease has been regarded as a single disease entity, however emergence of subtypes is challenging this premise, though presently there are more questions than answers. Researchers are studying neuroimages, genetic profiles and biomarkers in the brains, cerebrospinal fluid (CSF), and blood and skin of patients in the hope of identifying objective and quantifiable measures that will expand understanding of aetiology, improve evaluation of the efficacy of interventions and lead to improved treatments. This will hopefully support development of precision medicine so that specific interventions can be better targeted to individual needs.

But that is future aspiration. At present PD is a lifelong and dynamic condition. It can't be cured, and ongoing degeneration cannot be prevented, so change is inevitable. For now, the primary objective in all management is enabling individuals to adapt to this change, as it arises, and to maximise function.

But what does adaptation look like in practical terms and how does it translate to lived experience? The answer is not easily portrayed because it lies in the realm of subjectivity. The person best positioned to determine what adapting well looks like is the individual themselves. And herein lies one of the great challenges facing those seeking to develop health policy. There is no simple, neatly packaged, one size fits all solution. Although I have described my personal experiences with Parkinson's, it is only my journey and a partial one at that. Individuals may be connected by the common label of PD but there is significant diversity in their experience in terms of both symptoms and context. Symptoms impact the triad of physical, psychological and social function, and therefore establishing management plans for PD is not mass production but bespoke design. Even if two patients have the same clinical picture they may have different support networks, psychology and co-morbidity.

This inevitably creates problems for service design particularly in structures that are already under-resourced. If we really want to improve outcomes for those living with PD then the starting point must be the individual and they must remain at the heart of every management plan. It is not enough to embrace patient-centred personalised care as an ideal, we must strive until it is normative but to achieve this necessitates cultural change. It requires a national conversation in which embedded core societal beliefs need to be challenged to bring about reform. To put patients at the centre of their management requires a gradual dismantling of the status quo and has important ramifications for commissioning healthcare structures and service provision.

Managing a chronic progressive condition, which has more than forty symptoms and for which there is no disease-modifying treatment requires a very different model of care than conditions in which the aetiology and pathology are clearly understood and for which there are established interventions. It necessitates a model which is both holistic and collaborative.

At present we are largely managing the symptoms of disease rather than the pathology. Managing Parkinson's involves primarily managing the patient's lived experience, and this is vital to grasp. This is not a clinical context where the 'doctor always knows best.' The doctor will know best about some things such as medication and diagnosing complications, but that reflects only one dimension of management of lived experience. Understanding how the symptoms of PD integrate with the patients' psychology, social context, spirituality and the rest of their physical health is an important factor in achieving best outcomes. The patient and care partner voices must not only be heard but considered essential to any model of care, and it is important that dynamics of the healthcare relationships are such that the person with Parkinson's feels that the healthcare team has authorised them to take some control of their own Parkinson's management.

Any sense of pyramidal hierarchy within the healthcare team must also be dismantled. Each member of the multi-disciplinary team (MDT) involving clinicians, physiotherapists, occupational therapists, speech and language therapists, specialist nurses and dieticians, has an essential role in particular aspects of management and the keyworker at a given time will change with the condition.

Finally, when managing such a complex multisystem condition it is vital that specialisation does not occur at the cost of integration. Specialist input is imperative but must be accompanied by effective communication, evaluation of the big picture and collaborative working between all the different components to ensure an integrated outcome.

However reform must extend beyond healthcare structures to involve all of society. Currently much of the management in PD is reactive; responding to needs as they arise. In part this is driven by resources but there is also an absence of long-term strategy in policy making. Developing sustainable health economies in the future will, arguably, be best accomplished by promoting a shift towards a more proactive approach encouraging and enabling patients to take a more central role in their own management plans. For some patients this will be empowering, restoring a locus of control lost with the diagnosis, but for others it will escalate a sense of feeling overwhelmed. This is why there must be a holistic approach which takes account of all patient factors.

Resources are likely to remain stretched moving forward and will rightly be directed in the first instance to the vulnerable and those with the greatest needs.

But this will perpetuate systems which are reactive unless there is creativity, vision and innovation to establish new models of health and social care. In achieving this there must also be a clearer delineation between health and well-being, and an understanding that responsibility for the latter belongs to the whole of society including patients themselves. Employers, the charitable sector and community groups have a fundamental role in supporting aspects of management, as do family, friends, neighbours and members of the individual's community groups.

Until the advent of disease-modifying drugs, I believe there are three key ways to enable patients with PD manage their condition: educate, empower and equip.

To adapt means integrating into life something you didn't seek in the first place. No one desires the physical, mental or social impairment of function that accompany PD and until a cure is found there is a need to achieve balance between, on the one hand, doing everything possible to prevent change and maintain function, and, on the other, promoting change to enable adaptation.

To integrate a long-term condition relies on the individual's willingness to change – but not everyone wants to change. The ability to make this choice is enshrined in human rights. It may limit function and may be considered unwise by others but providing the individual has mental capacity that choice must be respected. However, disease factors must be assessed and high-quality information made available and accessible to patients to ensure that choice is informed. This is why medical and public education is so important. Individuals are more likely to engage and adapt if they are empowered, but they can only be empowered if in turn they are first educated to understand. This will involve signposting them to information at diagnosis that they can access when they are ready and absorb at their own pace. Information must be clear, accessible, reliable, evidence based and culturally sensitive. However, signposting will only be partially effective if it is not accompanied by follow-up and an opportunity to address questions that this reading will raise.

There must also be careful assessment to understand the factors affecting motivation. Despite being told my condition was at a mild stage and that I didn't need to be started on levodopa, I still felt shocked and numb. I was grieving and fearful of what the future would hold. Managing a condition in which the road ahead is unclear is not easy, and individuals may experience a breadth of varied emotions at different stages. They may be angry because of the diagnosis. They may feel frustrated that no one can give them concrete answers or despondent because scientific progress they read about doesn't seem to translate to their everyday experience. It is important to create safe environments for patients to talk about the impact of their diagnosis and address psychological aspects. This is very often managed informally by friends and family, but those who are isolated may require more intentional and structured support. This also needs to be reviewed intermittently as it will change with time and as the patient progresses through different stages of emotional processing.

Disease factors must also be carefully screened for. Depression, anxiety, apathy and executive dysfunction are all common in PD and will all influence both the desire and the ability to change by affecting motivation. Treating them not only brings symptom relief but can have broader effects on management of other symptoms. Treating depression improves energy and motivation, making physical activity easier which in turn helps motor function and mood. Finding and setting in motion these positively reinforcing spirals is the holy grail of medical management of PD.

But motivation alone is insufficient to cause change. It depends also upon opportunity. If we educate and empower patients but then fail to provide opportunity to equip it will certainly lead to individuals becoming stuck, disengaged and frustrated. Picture the scenario. A patient has read about how PD can impact their swallowing, learning this is a predictor of poor outcomes. But they have also read that there is a validated course which teaches exercises they can undertake to strengthen these muscles. They self-advocate at their next appointment to ask for a referral only to be informed the service is not available or cannot be funded. If we really desire to encourage proactivity and self-advocacy and establish true patient-centred care, it can't be done without reforming the way we commission health services. This is why broader national conversations are requiste if there is to be meaningful reform. Until this is achieved communication is key in managing patient expectations. When I had a physiotherapy assessment a few months after diagnosis I didn't feel it had addressed my needs. Years later I would realise that the physiotherapists were undertaking a 'Lindop Parkinson's Physiotherapy Assessment Scale (LPAS),' which is a validated tool to measure function. It is standard practice to establish a baseline, but as my walking and bed mobility were normal, I was quickly discharged. Physiotherapists do a fabulous job and make a massive difference to people living with Parkinson's, but with reflection I feel that with a more proactive model of care this could have been an opportunity to educate me about the importance of high-intensity exercise and help me to understand the importance of stretching, cardio, strength and balance work in maintaining my function.

I have considered how adaptability is one of the pillars of living well with any progressive condition, but the factors affecting it are not the same for everyone.

Some of these factors are societal. Improved access, legal frameworks such as the Equality Act and financial assistance in the form of benefits can all act positively and promote adaptability, on the other hand a lack of education, stigma and isolation impede it. However, it is important to avoid sweeping generalisations. Some patients applying for financial assistance can feel disincentivised to exercise for fear of being considered fraudulent. Collaborative working across different stakeholders and effective dialogue with patients and their care partners is essential if the societal barriers that remain are to be dismantled.

Other factors are personal and heavily influenced by personality, previous life experiences and disease factors. My previous life experiences of playing American football, growing up with an alcoholic father and changing career plans prepared me for what was to come with Parkinson's, as have aspects of my personality.

A third group are disease factors. Parkinson's is often described as a movement disorder, but that is only a partial representation. It is not just a movement disorder but a complex condition with non-motor symptoms that cause significant burden for both the individual and their carers. Some disease factors are fixed, such as the age that you were diagnosed or the side that your symptoms appeared on first. Right-sided symptoms in a right-handed person will be more impactful than if they had been on the left side and vice versa, but many fluctuate on a daily basis throughout the day complicating management.

Finally, there are healthcare factors such as timely access to specialist services, equity of access to centres of excellence and greater integration of neurology and psychiatry.

When we evaluate the number of variables which can differ between patients it is easy to see why there is a need for personalised care plans. The key to enabling patients to adapt well to their best life is to identify the roadblocks which exist for them and seek to remove as many as possible. For some it may be lack of access, for others it is pain, anxiety or discrimination in the workplace. However, despite the enormous diversity there are some common threads to every management plan: exercise, community and lifestyle.

Throughout this book I have considered the value of exercise and its importance in the management of PD. Research suggests that if you exercise for 30 minutes, three times a week, at about eighty percent of your maximum, the brain will start to make new functional connections. When I am at the gym and it's hard to keep persevering I close my eyes, listen to the music in my ear and envisage my neurons dancing to the beat.

I am certain that the evidence base for the benefits of exercise in PD will continue to expand and provide further clarity on the type and duration of exercise those with PD need to do, but in the meantime working out how to enable exercise at all, is key.

In the UK people spend a longer amount of time sitting on the toilet per week (3.5 hrs) than we do exercising (2.7 hrs). In 2021, 25.7% of people in England were deemed obese, having a BMI of over thirty or more, and ninety-five percent of people over the age of thirty never sprint again. If the general population isn't exercising, how much more difficult is it for a person with Parkinson's?

There are many factors affecting an individual's ability to exercise. These include time, priorities, motivation, fatigue, pain, finances, baseline fitness and stigma, and it is vital to understand these factors, to establish which can be addressed. But it is also important to realise that just as Parkinson's differs from person to person, so does the way that people exercise; it doesn't help to compare. Some people prefer to exercise on their own, others find group exercise more encouraging. Some will exercise standing, others will have to sit, while some like cycling, others walk. Ideally all those newly diagnosed with Parkinson's would be enabled to access a personalised physical exercise plan which considers age, pre-existing baseline fitness and the factors discussed above. Those who present with a prominent neuro-psychiatric non-motor symptom load such as depression, anxiety or apathy need more support at diagnosis from an exercise point of view. The key is to encourage patients to take the first steps. It doesn't need to be complex. Simple plans with what is familiar is a good starting point.

There is a wealth of helpful information based on the World Health Organisation's (WHO) Guidelines on Physical Activity and Sedentary Behaviour. The Parkinson's Excellence Network Exercise Hub, a group of specialist physiotherapists in the UK, have produced guidance about the type and amount of exercise that is recommended, and all charities do a good job of promoting, educating and providing online exercise resources.

It is also important to encourage individuals to connect with others. No one has unwavering motivation or can keep going all the time. But everyone's care circle will look different. There are no hard and fast rules. I find it helpful to surround myself with like-minded people who encourage and keep me stubbornly positive, but I'm also increasingly aware of the need for balance and to have those who are not afraid to challenge and prevent me becoming too blinkered. My key point is that it's hard to do it alone: this is a long journey.

Finally, there are important proactive lifestyle choices everyone can make. These include maintaining hydration, eating a healthy diet and avoiding high protein loads, especially around doses, keeping bowels moving regularly and proactively looking after bone strength to prevent fractures.

The year after I was diagnosed, we were fortunate to spend a week on a cruise of the Caribbean. During one of the 'days at sea' I escaped the crowds and entertainment to sit for an hour on the balcony. In every direction the horizon was a blue glassy stillness, so much so, it was difficult to distinguish the sea from the sky. And yet the appearance was deceptive for the sea was in perpetual motion. PD is a condition which is constantly evolving. The goal of management is to find calm waters where this perpetual motion goes almost unnoticed day by day. It is vital to prepare for stormy weather which will inevitably arise by implementing measures: a captain with knowledge, instruments to change course, stabilisers to add ballast and the security of a harbour if needed. I believe that this will be best achieved when as a society we educate, empower and equip individuals through holistic person-centred healthcare enabling them to live their best life.

Epilogue

As I finish writing nearly a year since I started, the dawn chorus is singing again, but daylight hasn't appeared as yet. These words were some of the easiest and yet the hardest to write in the quietness at the start of the day, I knew what I wanted to say but it took a while to get them down on paper. I needed time and this was when I still had the most.

This book has helped me process many life experiences and I am grateful to have been able to do that. As I was sitting thinking I kept being taken back to words that my dad used to say as he battled his alcohol addiction. They are known as the Serenity Prayer.

'God grant me the serenity to accept the things I cannot change. Courage to change the things I can, and the wisdom to know the difference.'

These words accept, courage and wisdom are all needed when living with a Parkinson's diagnosis as we wrestle with its impact over time. But it is the word serenity that stands out as I cannot do it with a calmness and an inner peace on my own strength, I need help. Parkinson's is ever changing I don't know how I will be feeling throughout each day, but the one constant in all of this one that doesn't change is a loving God. One who provides the daily grace needed to get through the day. This has given me the strength to get up every morning and keep going.

I don't know what the future holds; no one does. But I do know that my time here on earth is a small chunk of my life and that helps me to frame and endure it. When I look up to the heavenly sky, there is a day coming when I will have a fully functioning substantia nigra. Until then I close my eyes and long for the day when all of my neurons will dance once again.

DOI: 10.1201/9781003600671-21

End Notes

THE LONG WALK

Goddard JF. 2008. *The Palace on the Hill.* [online]. Available from https://www.leicester
mercury.co.uk/news/history/hospital-affectionately-know-the-palace-1776916 [Accessed
29 May 2024]

SIMPLY COMPLEX

Giroux M, Farris S, Bas B. 2012. *Every Victory Counts.* [online]. Available from https://
davisphinneyfoundation.org/every-victory-counts-manual/ [Accessed 29 May 2024]
The Davis Phinney Foundation. 2014. *The Parkinson's You Don't See: Cognitive and Non-Motor
Symptoms.* [online]. Available from https://www.youtube.com/watch?v=S2LP_5PC9LU
[Accessed 30 May 2024]

THIS BIKE IS ON ME

Parkinson's UK Physical Activity and Exercise. 2024. [online]. Available from https://www.
parkinsons.org.uk/information-and-support/physical-activity-and-exercise?utm_
source=google&utm_medium=cpc&utm_campaign=&utm_term=parkinson%27s%20
exercises&utm_content=&gad_source=1&gclid=Cj0KCQiA4-y8BhC3ARIsAHmjC_
EdItxlTJ2oieIADURNkE0f5WIL-1q [Accessed 3 June 2024]
World Health Organisations (WHO). 2020. *Guidelines on Physical Activity and
Sedentary Behaviour.* [online]. Available from https://www.who.int/publications/i/
item/9789240015128 [Accessed 2 June 2024]

MUSCLE MEMORY

Toth A. 2022. *The Science behind Muscle Memory.* [online]. Available from https://scopeblog.
stanford.edu/2022/07/15/the-science-behind-muscle-memory/ [Accessed 8 June 2024]

THE ED WITH PD

Radad K, Moldzio R, Krewenka C, Kranner B, Rausch WD. 2023. *Pathophysiology of Non-
motor Signs in Parkinson's Disease: Some Recent Updating with Brief Presentation.*
[online]. Available from https://pmc.ncbi.nlm.nih.gov/articles/PMC6986277/ [Accessed
10 June 2024]
Ranijbar-Slamloo Y, Fazlali Z. 2020. *Dopamine and Noradrenaline in the Brain; Overlapping or
Dissociate Functions?* [online]. Available from https://www.explorationpub.com/Journals/
ent/Article/100436#:~:text=Non%2Dmotor%20signs%20in%20PD,In%20contrast
%20to&text=They%20are%20attributed%20to%20the,and%20autonomic%20dys
functions%20%5B8%5D [Accessed 12 June 2024]

CONNECTIONS AND COPING

Brody J. 2011. *Marching through Life with Parkinson's*. [online]. Available from https://www.nytimes.com/2011/06/14/health/14brody.html [Accessed 14 July 2024]

Galloway B. 2015. *One to Punch*. [online]. Available from https://www.parkinsonsmorethanmotion.com/story/one-two-punch [Accessed 14 July 2024]

KYOTO

English: My Dad His Parkinson's through My 9-year-old Eyes. 2018. [online]. Available from https://www.youtube.com/watch?v=F0WzJWjqcD0 [Accessed 31 January 2025] and https://www.jonnyacheson.com

Galloway B. 2016. *Spotlight on Soania Mathur (USA)*. [online]. Available from https://www.ucb.com/patients/Life-stories/parkinsons-disease/Soania [Accessed 15 July 2024]

WhenLife Gives You Parkinson's Podcast. 2018. [online]. Available from https://www.curiouscast.ca/podcast/160/when-life-gives-you-parkinsons/ [Accessed 17 July]

COMMUNITY

Landowski L. 2021. *Finding That Connection© – Neurons Connecting to One Another in a Petri Dish – Growth Cones*. [online]. Available from https://www.youtube.com/watch?v=Rvmvt7gscIM [Accessed 3 August 2024]

Lees AJ. 1992. *When Did Ray Kennedy's Parkinson's Disease Begin?* [online]. Movement Disorders. Available from Movement Disorders. Available from https://pubmed.ncbi.nlm.nih.gov/1584235/ [Accessed 4 August 2024]

COVID

UK Government. 2021. *COVID-19: Guidance for People Whose Immune System Means They Are at Higher Risk*. [online]. Available from https://www.gov.uk/government/publications/covid-19-guidance-for-people-whose-immune-system-means-they-are-at-higher-risk [Accessed 16 August 2024]

HEALTHCARE PROFESSIONALS WITH PARKINSON'S

All the Same but Different. 2022. [online]. Available from https://www.youtube.com/watch?v=soxn8soxTmY [Accessed 31 January 2025]

Connecting through Care: The Inside Job. 2021. [online]. Available from https://www.youtube.com/watch?v=8pcWSmZNqdk [Accessed 31 January 2025]

LA SAGRADA FAMILIA

WPC. 2023. *What Do Subtypes Mean for People with Parkinson's*. [online]. Available from https://www.youtube.com/watch?v=_A1rYi4h2QI [Accessed 31 January 2025]

TIME CRITICAL MEDICATION

HSJ Patient Safety Awards. 2023. *Patient Involvement in Safety Award.* [online]. Available from https://www.hsj.co.uk/hsj-patient-safety-awards-2023-patient-involvement-in-safety-award/7035511.article [Accessed 31 January 2025]

McLeod, A. *100,000 Parkinson's Medication Errors Each Year in Scotland's Hospitals.* [online]. Available from https://www.alliance-scotland.org.uk/blog/opinion/100000-parkinsons-medication-errors-each-year-in-scotlands-hospitals/ [Accessed 31 January 2025]

NHS England. 2023. *The National Patient Safety Improvement Programmes.* [online]. Available from https://www.england.nhs.uk/patient-safety/patient-safety-improvement-programmes/#national-patient-safety-improvement-programme [Accessed 31 January 2025]

Parkinson's UK. 2019. *Get It on Time Report.* [online]. Available from https://www.parkinsons.org.uk/sites/default/files/2019-10/CS3380%20Get%20it%20on%20Time%20Report%20A4%20final%2026.09.2019-compressed%20%281%29.pdf [Accessed 31 January 2025]

Parkinson's UK. 2023. *Every Minute Counts Time Critical Parkinson's Medication on Time, Every Time.* [online]. Available from https://www.parkinsons.org.uk/sites/default/files/2023-09/CS4006%20Get%20it%20on%20time%20policy%20report_Web%20Version.pdf [Accessed 31 January 2025]

The Royal College Of Emergency Medicine. 2023. *EM Consultant's Very Personal Commitment to RCEM's Latest Quality Improvement Programme.* [online]. Available from https://rcem.ac.uk/consultants-commitment-to-latest-rcem-qip/ [Accessed 31 January 2025].

CO-MORBIDITIES

British Heart Foundation. 2025. *Northern Ireland Factsheet.* [online]. Available from https://www.bhf.org.uk/-/media/files/for-professionals/research/heart-statistics/bhf-cvd-statistics-northern-ireland-factsheet.pdf?rev=2250381cc530479ebe843015b4d0cd93&hash=354E5F29900D6ABDB067300A80167D44 [Accessed 1 February 2025]

Kaplan H et al. 2017. Coronary atherosclerosis in indigenous South American Tsimané: A cross-sectional cohort study. *The Lancet.* [online]. Available from https://thelancet.com/journals/lancet/article/PllS0140-6736(17)30752-3/abstract [Accessed 31 January 2025]

ENABLING NOT DISABLING

Johansson M et al. 2002. *Aerobic Exercise Alters Brain Function and Structure in Parkinson's Disease: A Randomized Controlled Trial.* [online]. Available from Annals of Neurology https://pubmed.ncbi.nlm.nih.gov/34951063/ [Accessed 4 February 2025]

Official Statistics, National Statistics, Survey. 2017. *Accredited Official Statistics.* [online]. Health Survey for England, 2021 part 1. Available from https://digital.nhs.uk/data-and-information/publications/statistical/health-survey-for-england/2021/overweight-and-obesity-in-adults [Accessed 5 February 2025]

Oliver D. 2017. *People in the UK Spend More Time on the Toilet Than Exercising.* [online]. Available from https://www,health.usnews.com/wellness/health-buzz/articles/2017-09-26/people-in-the-uk-spend-more-time-on-the-toilet-than-exercising [Accessed 7 February 2025]

Appendix 1

My Dad: His Parkinson's through My Nine-Year-Old Eyes Script

Hi, I'm nine years old and I love telling stories.

This is my dad, he always seemed to be tired and he would even fall asleep before I went to bed.

My Dad told me he was also tired in work. I thought he must be very busy.

We went to London on holidays but he didn't like being in large crowds.

My Dad kept tripping and found it hard walking around London all day.

We had to come home early I was sad as I wanted to see the big glass tower.

I also noticed that my dad was very quiet at teatime, he didn't talk a lot and stopped telling jokes.

One day my dad realised that he couldn't do the change the lightbulb dance because his left wrist wouldn't move quickly.

My Dad told my Mum that his left arm started to shake when he was driving to work and he couldn't stop it.

My Dad and Mum decided to go to the doctor in our village, when I was at school.

Then they had to go to the hospital and see a special doctor. My Dad said he was nervous, so did my Mum.

My Dad concentrated hard not to trip when he had to walk but the doctor said he didn't swing his left arm very much.

When my dad told us that evening that he had Parkinson's Disease, we all had a family hug.

My Dad said that he didn't have enough chemicals in a part of his brain that helped him move and be himself. It begins with a 'D.'

So, what's it like having a dad with Parkinson's?

I know that my dad needs to exercise a lot.

I know my dad doesn't like to be rushed, I'm working on that.

Somedays when he gets home from work, he needs to rest so I get him to play sleeping lions instead of running games outside.

When my dad is tired, he walks into door frames. I did the same yesterday to make him feel better.

Sometimes my dad just likes to have quiet, I find this hard.

When my dad drops plates in the kitchen I help him.

I know that my dad loves me and we have lots of fun. He has even started telling jokes again.

I do wonder what caused my Dad's Parkinson's. Hopefully one day someone will find out.

The End.

Appendix 2

Time Critical Medications: Ten Recommendations for Hospitals

1. Parkinson's medication is Time Critical Medication. Time Critical Medications must be given within thirty minutes of when they are due, highlighted as a risk to patient safety and added to every hospital risk register. Compliance is audited and any dose over thirty minutes should be reported as an adverse event.

2. All hospital staff are made aware of Time Critical Medication. Make this three-minute video, *Time Matters: It's Critical*, mandatory viewing for all staff.

3. Hospitals identify which staff are to undertake further Parkinson's medication training. Recommended online training courses are available via the Parkinson's Excellence Network's Learning Hub:
   a. Parkinson's UK fifteen-minute Educational Video
   b. Parkinson's UK Medication Educational Module produced by Lancashire Teaching Hospitals
   c. Parkinson's medication for staff who don't administer medications

4. Hospitals develop, maintain and update a self-administration policy for patients who can administer their own medication. The policy should be reviewed regularly.

5. Hospitals identify all patients on Time Critical Medication when they arrive in the Emergency Department (ED) or through an elective or emergency admissions unit.

6. EDs and admissions units develop and update an agreed list of Time Critical Medication visible to patients when they arrive so they feel empowered to inform staff that they take Time Critical Medication. For elective admissions, people with Parkinson's will have prepared themselves. Parkinson's UK Guidance.

7. Hospitals have a designated pharmacist who is responsible for ordering and stocking the Time Critical Medications in the ED and on appropriate admissions units and wards to ensure they are always available.

8. Where appropriate, the prescribing of a patient's Time Critical Medication should reflect their normal daily schedule and should continue during the full admission period. Hospital systems, including electronic prescribing where available, should be maximised to support this.

9   Ensure that hospitals have a Standard Operating Procedure/guideline for all Time Critical Medication, including patients who are nil by mouth (NBM) or require a nasogastric (NG) tube. This should signpost to one of the NBM medication calculators.

10 Ensure hospitals devise and implement a system so that staff can administer all Time Critical Medications outside of normal medication rounds if self-administration is not appropriate.

For Product Safety Concerns and Information please contact our EU
representative GPSR@taylorandfrancis.com
Taylor & Francis Verlag GmbH, Kaufingerstraße 24, 80331 München, Germany

9 7 8 1 0 3 2 9 8 9 9 9 7 6